The International Behavioural and Social Sciences Library

LEAVING RESIDENTIAL CARE

TAVISTOCK

The International Behavioural and Social Sciences Library

HEALTH & SOCIETY
In 12 Volumes

I	Industrial Organizations and Health
	Edited by Frank Baker, et al.
II	Six Minutes for the Patient
	Edited by Enid Balint and J S Norell
III	A Study of Doctors
	Michael Balint, et al.
IV	Treatment or Diagnosis
	Michael Balint, et al.
V	Admission to Residential Care
	Paul Brearley
VI	Leaving Residential Care
	Paul Brearley
VII	Culture, Health and Disease
	Margaret Read
VIII	Management in the Social and Safety Services
	Edited by W D Reekie and Norman C Hunt
IX	Contemporary Community
	Jacqueline Scherer
X	Towards Community Mental Health
	Edited by John D Sutherland
XI	An Introduction to Medical Sociology
	Edited by David Tuckett
XII	Open Employment After Mental Illness
	Nancy Wansbrough and Philip Cooper

LEAVING RESIDENTIAL CARE

PAUL BREARLEY
WITH JIM BLACK, PENNY GUTRIDGE,
GWYNETH ROBERTS AND ELIZABETH
TARRAN

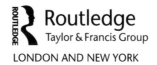

Routledge
Taylor & Francis Group
LONDON AND NEW YORK

First published in 1982 by
Tavistock Publications Limited

Published in 2001 by
Routledge
2 Park Square, Milton Park, Abingdon, Oxfordshire OX14 4RN
711 Third Avenue, New York, NY 10017

First issued in paperback 2014

Routledge is an imprint of the Taylor and Francis Group, an informa business

© 1982 P Brearley, J Black, P Gutridge, G Roberts and E
Tarran

British Library Cataloguing in Publication Data
A CIP catalogue record for this book
is available from the British Library

Leaving Residential Care
ISBN 0-415-26429-4
Health & Society: 12 Volumes
ISBN 0-415-26509-6
The International Behavioural and Social Sciences Library
112 Volumes
ISBN 0-415-25670-4

ISBN 13: 978-1-138-86742-0 (pbk)
ISBN 13: 978-0-415-26429-7 (hbk)

Leaving Residential Care

Paul Brearley,

WITH
*Jim Black, Penny Gutridge,
Gwyneth Roberts, and Elizabeth Tarran*

TAVISTOCK PUBLICATIONS
LONDON AND NEW YORK

First published in 1982 by
Tavistock Publications Ltd
2 Park Square, Milton Park,
Abingdon, Oxon, OX14 4RN
Published in the USA by
Tavistock Publications
in association with Routledge.
270 Madison Ave,
New York NY 10016
© 1982 P. Brearley, J. Black,
P. Gutridge, G. Roberts, and
E. Tarran
Typeset in Great Britain by
Scarborough Typesetting Services

British Library Cataloguing in
Publication Data

Brearley, Paul
Leaving residential
care.—(Residential social work)
1. Institutional care—Great Britain
2. Inmates of institutions—Great
Britain
I. Title   II. Series
361'.05   HV245
ISBN 0–422–77930–X Pbk

Library of Congress Cataloguing in
Publication Data

Brearley, C. Paul.
Leaving residential care.
(Social science paperbacks)
Bibliography: p.
Includes indexes.
1. Medical social work.
2. Rehabilitation.
I. Black, Jim. II. Title. III. Series.
HV687.B73 1982   362'.0425
82–7980   AACR2
ISBN 0–422–77930–X (pbk.)

Contents

General Editor's Foreword   vi

PART ONE
Introduction   *Paul Brearley*   3
1   The Experience and Process of Leaving
    Paul Brearley   11
2   Legal Aspects   *Gwyneth Roberts*   35

PART TWO
Introduction   *Paul Brearley*   59
3   Children   *Penny Gutridge*   63
4   Handicapped Children   *Elizabeth Tarran*   94
5   The Elderly   *Paul Brearley*   117
6   Mental Hospitals   *Jim Black*   146
    Conclusion   *Paul Brearley*   173
    References   179
    Name Index   192
    Subject Index   196

General Editor's Foreword

Residential social work has sometimes been described as a 'people-processing system' — a somewhat callous and mechanistic definition, it is true, but one which serves to highlight the fact that residential care is a process which, to use a similarly mechanistic phrase, has an 'end-product'. As the authors of this book say, it is surprising that little attention has been paid either to the beginning of this process or to its end, and, in particular, that the latter seems to have been considered as a natural, and therefore undesigned, outcome of what has gone before.

Surprise at this state of affairs is appropriate because logically the whole process of residential care can be seen as moving towards a return to a so-called 'normal' form of existence in the community. After careful consideration, what other criteria of success are available to us other than that such a transfer has been successfully effected for the majority of those subjected to the care process? Of course methods of measuring the rate or even the degree of success are very hard to devise and even harder to put into practice. Most practitioners and administrators are content to accept as an effective measure of success the simple fact of no re-entry by discharged clients into the system. For the more particular this would have to be expanded to no re-entry into any other similar system.

If the logical outcome of the process called residential care is the return of those cared for to the community, then the whole process should not only be geared to that end, but every part of the process should contribute to it and be planned and executed to achieve it. This is the concept of continuity of care which the authors are at great pains to present here, showing that the planning for discharge, for leaving, is crucial not only to the final success of residential care but also to its performance.

The problems attendant upon such planning are many, and

often revolve around the lack of hard information, adequate resources, and appropriate skills. No less important are those ubiquitous problems connected with the transfer of people from encapsulating and supportive environments into the community at large. The process of leaving care is often a major life transition and must rank fairly high on the scale of stress factors which act cumulatively to reduce the level of functioning of those subjected to them. This reduction of functional normality cannot be prevented, but its effects can be anticipated and allowed for, and the outcome substantially ameliorated. Thus the important measure following recognition of the possibility of stress is preparation which discusses the possible effects, releases methods of coping, and supplies contacts with possible support systems.

As in their previous text in this series, *Admission to Residential Care*, the authors have considered the legal aspects of the process they are examining. The law often specifies that, given certain conditions, certain procedures are appropriate; sometimes it says when, sometimes even why, but seldom if ever does it say how. It is exactly this vexed question of how appropriate actions may be performed which often causes the greatest headaches for practitioners, and it is just such problems and their possible solutions which are addressed by the authors with reference to children, the mentally ill, and the elderly.

In this area of highly personal difficulties prescription is too narrow a form of help. Therefore, what is offered is a set of general ideas related to the problem of leaving care which cover the essential principles that are known. On the basis of this generalized information adaptations to fit each individual circumstance can be contrived on a sound basis and with a good prospect of success.

The authors encourage practitioners to review those constraints in the care process which have been accepted traditionally and regarded as immovable, or nearly so, such as the high improbability that old people admitted to care will ever be discharged back into society with some qualified degree of independence. They argue that possibilities are sometimes not explored, not because they do not exist, but more often because it has become accepted practice to believe that they are not possibilities in any 'real' sense at all, even though such beliefs have not been properly tested.

The emotional factors of leaving care, such as 'separation anxieties' are given an airing here as are traditionally accepted (by the carers) attitudes amongst those cared for, for example that they will see care as a dubious, frustrating, and unrewarding experience, from which release and return to freedom cannot come too soon. What little evidence we have shows such attitudes to be uncommon and even when they do exist to be very rarely free of ambivalence.

All in all this brief text lets some healthy gusts of fresh air into a part of the process of care that has received far too little consideration and, as in their previous book, the authors have contributed a worthwhile addition to the all too scanty literature designed for the practitioners of residential care.

TOM DOUGLAS
February 1982

Part One

Introduction   *Paul Brearley*

This book is intended as a companion volume to our earlier collection of essays, which appeared in this series as *Admission to
Residential Care* (Brearley *et al.* 1980). We began that earlier
work with an enthusiasm that was encouraged by the knowledge
that there was relatively little substantial written material on the
subject of admission to residential living, in spite of the fact that
most social workers are frequently involved in the admission
process. In developing the ideas and material we became aware
of an even more striking gap in the general literature available
about leaving residential care. What follows, therefore, is an
attempt to draw together the existing writings about social work
practice with a variety of different groups of people in care in
the light of our own experiences. Much of the existing material
is anecdotal, or in the form of exhortations or generalized prescriptions. Our intention is to develop common themes around
which emerge approaches to good practice which we believe can
be applied to the range of contexts presented.

   In our previous book four main themes were identified. First,
people are admitted to care because they are vulnerable in their
living situation: they are at risk. However, since admission to
care itself involves specific hazards, and living in care involves
exposure to further hazards, people should ideally only enter
care if it is clear that the potential benefits outweigh the
potential disadvantages. Second, admission to residential care
can be viewed as a process of change through time which moves
from the recognition of hazards or potential dangers, through a
decision on action, preparation, and transfer, to arrival and
settling in. This process is similar for a range of settings and
types of residential care, although the decisions and approaches
made within and in association with the process are affected by
various factors, and the time-span and emphases within the

process will also vary. Third, good practice in relation to the residential setting has been closely linked with the importance of creating options. Choice is increasingly being seen as an essential right of the individual in care, but one which must be exercised responsibly: choice and responsibility are inextricably linked. Fourth, and this is linked to the previous theme, information and communication are also central to good practice. It is important that people should be able to choose the kind of life they wish to lead within the limits of their environment and they should therefore clearly understand what is available, and be helped to select where necessary. Communication is also an essential factor in developing working relationships between groups of workers involved in using residential resources or in working with the residential setting.

One task of this book will be to pursue these themes as they relate to the experience of leaving care. The concepts of risk and vulnerability, of choice and responsibility, and of information and communication all have a place in the consideration of the experience of the process of entering, living in, and leaving the residential setting. There are, of course, some very obvious differences between entering and leaving residential care. However well the individual has been prepared for admission, the time between making the decision to enter care and the actual transition is unlikely to be as long for the great majority of people as the time available to anticipate leaving care. The possibility for each experience to be a major life event with a lasting impact exists but the period for preparation, apprehension, or expectation when leaving care is likely to be much longer. One reason for this is that a high proportion of admissions take place rapidly as an urgent and immediate response to an emergency: leaving care is unlikely to happen as an emergency. Similarly, admission is relatively frequently a consequence of compulsory action: leaving care may be the consequence of the termination or lapse of compulsory powers, and the issues are correspondingly different.

Although it will be appropriate to develop some issues from the discussion of admission to care, the experience of admission is clearly very different from that of leaving care and a number of new perspectives must be considered. It is particularly important to clarify the concept of 'care' in this context. Care is a word that is used to describe a feeling experienced by some people for or towards others, but it is also used to refer to actions taken by some for others. More specifically, the concept of care refers to the provision of formal services by agencies to meet the needs of individuals. 'Leaving care' refers to broader issues than solely moving from a residential setting. Many children who are regarded as being in care, for example, live with foster parents and, even if subject to a care order, many remain with their own parents. Of the 100,000 children in care in England and Wales in 1978, about one third were boarded out and almost one in five (18,900) were in the charge of a parent, guardian, relative, or friend (Central Statistical Office 1981). The entry to the status 'in care' does not, therefore, necessarily involve environmental change and it is possible to 'leave care' in the sense of giving up the status 'in care' without any change of environment. There is a difference between leaving care which involves only a *change of status* and the experience of leaving care which also involves a *change of environment*. This book is mainly concerned with the second of these, with those clients who are involved in moving from one environment to another. It is therefore primarily about people leaving residential environments.

However, we do not feel that a consideration of those institutional environments most commonly referred to as 'residential care' will present a full picture. It is also necessary to consider the experience of leaving other forms of institutional living. Social workers are involved with people who leave residential homes for children, the disabled, and sometimes (though less commonly), the elderly, but they are also involved organizationally in rather different ways with people leaving hospitals, prisons, hostels for the homeless, etc. In addition it must be recognized that not all people who leave enclosed institutional living environments return immediately to independent life in the community. Many people move to hostels, or forms of 'half-way houses', or simply move from one institution to another. In presenting a full consideration of the issues involved, it will be necessary to take account of the fact that people leave a wide variety of institutions and move to an equal variety of alternative living situations, ranging from enclosed prisons to open and independent community life.

The first chapter will set out general basic issues relating to the experience of leaving the institutional environment and sub-sequent chapters will develop the ideas in relation to specific contexts and client groups. It is our belief that moving from an enclosed living situation creates similar feelings and problems for everyone. Although it is obvious that a middle-aged man released from hospital, or perhaps from prison, will have many needs, expectations, and feelings different from those of an adolescent leaving a local authority children's home, we believe there are sufficient similarities to justify a common base for discussion of approaches to good social work practice.

POLICY AND PRIORITIES

In a government statement on priorities for the Health and Personal Social Services in 1981 it was suggested that, 'It has been a major policy objective for many years to foster and develop community care for the main client groups – elderly, mentally ill, mentally handicapped and disabled people, and children.' It is clear that the expression 'community care' is used to distinguish residential care as a separate provision. The statement continues: 'the specific objectives of community care policies are different for the different client groups, but the general aim is to maintain a person's link with family and friends and normal life, and to offer the support that meets his or her particular needs' (DHSS 1981a:21). These comments provide a summary of the position which has been adopted for many years in relation to all client groups. There is a general assumption that life in an institutional or residential situation is less desirable than life in other community settings, and that efforts should be directed towards preventing admission or, failing that, to returning people to the community. As an earlier government discussion document about the needs of older people puts it: 'we have aimed to keep old people active and independent in their own home. And where they have had to go into hospital, to get them back into their own home as soon as possible' (DHSS/Welsh Office 1978:4).

This view of residential care as a last resort has been bound up with the low status and frequently noted professional isolation of residential workers. Yet the fact remains that substantial numbers of people do spend time in institutional or residential situations, many of them for a considerable number of years. In 1978 there were just over 100,000 children in care in England and Wales (compared with a figure of 62,200 in 1961). Of these some 40,000 were in forms of institutional accommodation. The average daily UK population in prisons and in custody in 1979 included 48,000 men and 1,700 women. In psychiatric hospitals in the UK the average daily number of mental illness beds in use in 1978 was 102,700 and of mental handicap beds was 56,800. Residential accommodation was provided for almost 170,000 elderly people in local authority, voluntary, and private accommodation in the UK in 1978 (Central Statistical Office 1981). Clearly very large numbers of people are experiencing some form of institutional living at any moment in time.

The extent of this experience is emphasized in the light of figures for receptions and discharge from various forms of institutional provision. In 1979, for instance, 163,300 people were received into custody and the prison system in the UK, compared with the average daily population of about 50,000. In 1978 there were 221,400 deaths or discharges from mental illness beds and a further 23,600 from mental handicap beds in the UK (Central Statistical Office 1981). In England, in 1977, 96,200 children were in care, 49,600 were admitted to care, and almost 47,000 went out of care (DHSS 1978a). There is, in other words, not only a very large institutional population, but a substantial 'throughput' of people into and out of the various systems. The numbers of people encountering institutional life are therefore higher than any snapshot view of the figures might suggest.

Although policy statements do emphasize the desirability of

community care it is difficult to escape the weight of evidence that residential care is an inevitable component of the total range of services, and most commentators add a sometimes reluctant rider to this effect to their prescriptions for community care. David Ennals has summarized this more positively than most:

'The unique feature of the residential setting is that it can provide a focus for specialist services and skills combined with continuous personal and social care. The resource is too costly and the skills too scarce to provide them as substitutes for equally effective and cheaper services. But residential care will continue to provide the only satisfactory answer to particular combinations of needs'

(Ennals 1978:15)

It must be recognized that for some people residential or institutional care is the best available solution at a particular time in their lives. The priority statement quoted at the beginning of this section acknowledges this in commenting on the number of children in local authority care: 'While some of these children are best cared for in residential homes, far more of them could benefit from living in a family environment with foster parents' (DHSS 1981a:38). Similarly, although with a different emphasis, the White Paper on services for the elderly notes that 'whatever success is achieved in improving community care there will always be a significant minority of elderly people who cannot continue to live in their own homes' (DHSS/Scottish, Welsh and NI Offices 1981:44).

The overwhelming trend in policy statements about virtually all groups is to stress the importance of community living and the 'last resort' or temporary nature of institutional care. However even the general figures given here amply illustrate the absurdity of ignoring the residential sector, which is a major element in health and social service provision as well as custodial provision. The particular significance of such provision lies not only in its impact on the lives of large numbers of people but also in the substantial cost of providing institutions. This combination of a continual questioning of the appropriateness of institutional provision (and its considerable economic cost), taken together with the substantial numbers of people living in institutions, must underline the importance of the process of leaving the institutional system. The experience of leaving (or of discharge, or release) is encountered by many people, and although the great majority will not require social work help many do need such help. It is therefore particularly surprising that more has not been written about social work practice in this context.

RISK AND VULNERABILITY

In our previous book (Brearley *et al.* 1980) we have set out a structure for thinking about the analysis of the risks involved in social work situations. It is not necessary to repeat that discussion here but the reader is recommended to consider that account since some of the elements outlined will be incorporated in the subsequent discussion. Essentially, it must be recognized that involvement in the lives of others requires taking risks, and since by definition the people who enter residential care are vulnerable, this is particularly true of social work with this group.

The concept of risk involves two elements: that of loss, or chance of loss, and that of probability or possibility. Social work in risk situations is therefore concerned with values (and a balancing of potential losses and potential gains) and with prediction (making decisions about expected outcomes). Decision-making and action about leaving institutional care does involve making decisions about risks. Change creates hazards and potential dangers, and good preparation, planning, and support can help to reduce these hazards and dangers. Effective management of the process of leaving rests on detailed assessment, including assessment and evaluation of the risks involved.

The rest of this book will be concerned with exploring the issues involved in helping people to move through and out of a variety of forms of institutional living. The first two chapters set out general issues: first, in relation to common elements of the process of leaving; and, second, in relation to legal aspects of that process. Social workers now require an extensive knowledge of complex legal provisions and only the most commonly encountered situations are explored here. In the second part of the book the needs of three groups – children, children with handicaps, and older people – are discussed to illustrate some of the issues which arise in those situations which are most easily recognized as 'residential care'. Substantial numbers of children and of older people are cared for in residential homes in which the primary tasks of providing for the everyday needs for food, warmth, comfort, safety, etc. are very closely bound up with assumptions about the need for personal growth, independence, and integrity. In such homes there is an acceptance of the centrality of social work. In other institutions the social work role is much more obviously secondary to the main purpose of the establishment (although not necessarily secondary to the lives of many of the individuals who live there), and in the final chapter we therefore consider the issues which can arise through the example of social work in psychiatric hospitals.

We believe that it is important to develop common themes in social work and to look for ways of using knowledge which has proved helpful in one situation in other contexts. One consequence of taking the process of leaving care as the main theme of this discussion is that there is relatively little space to develop discussion of specific aspects of the needs of each group or situation that we have chosen to include, and wherever possible we have included reference to additional relevant reading.

1 The Experience and Process of Leaving *Paul Brearley*

A considerable number of factors play their part in determining how the individual experiences the end of a stay in an institution: whether admission was initially for protection or for treatment, for instance, or rehabilitation, or containment, restriction, or imprisonment. Similarly, the length of stay will be influential: leaving psychiatric hospital after a few days of enforced observation and treatment will be a very different experience from leaving a children's home after several years having established a close relationship with residential staff. Before proceeding to a more general discussion we will look at some insights into this experience from personal records and statements, and from case studies. The great majority of these are from the child care setting, and it is possible to distinguish reflections on the anticipation of leaving from records of the actual separation and the readjustment period.

Ollivant (1979:72), when working as a youth worker, recalled his own experience in care:

'No-one spoke to me specifically about leaving care so I kept pushing it to the back of my mind, although the inevitable was always there. At 15, I was fairly well settled. I was living with people who were genuinely concerned about me and who I had come to trust and respect, probably for the first time in my life. I would never have admitted it at the time but the thought of leaving scared me stiff.'

This is echoed by Leslie Thomas, author of several popular novels, writing about a similar time in his own life:

'And all the time, as you grew from being just a boy, you made plans for the time when you went through the gate for the last time and the Outside was waiting. Sometimes they were more fears than plans. Fears that life on your own would be too difficult, that people out there would stare.'

(Thomas 1967:150)

The most conspicuous theme in all the accounts is ambivalence. Many people describe feelings of expectation and anticipation but these are associated with feelings of anxiety and apprehension at the realistic, or imagined, problems which can be expected. This is not restricted to children: staff too will have mixed feelings. A study of the experience of being released from prison quotes accounts which bear striking similarities to those of children: 'a lot will be looking forward to coming out, but it's a waste of time: there are more problems out here' (Corden *et al.* 1978:7).

There is, of course, a difference between the time of anticipating leaving, which seems to be characterized by some degree of ambivalence for most commentators, and the reality of the experience. The study of released prisoners quotes contrasting accounts:

'It's the first time I've been inside. I did not imagine it would be as bad as this coming out: financially it's been terrible − I can't go anywhere − I have no clothes, etc. Unless I get a job, there's no way out − I feel like a tramp . . . in many ways you're better off inside − at least you've got a bed there.'

'It's been all right − the same as any other month really, as I expected it would be. It seems a long time ago since I was inside . . . a job would have made a difference, but there haven't been any real financial problems.'

(Corden *et al.* 1978:7)

Once again the ambivalence is apparent: institutional living provides an element of familiarity, security, or predictability and leaving that familiar environment involves encountering a range of practical problems and demands. A small study of young people who had recently left residential care identifies very similar factors: the author notes a large gap between being in care and being in the community and quotes some of his respondents:

'It's too much all at once.'

'There seemed to be nothing left. I felt lost.'

'I really wanted to move out and do things for myself but when I did I felt lost.'

(Godek 1977:36)

This author stresses the experience of loss and being alone at the time of leaving care and also notes that these changes occur when the problems of adolescence are at their height. It should be remembered that the reasons which bring some people into institutions can create an increased vulnerability to the impact of change.

The lack of planning and preparation is also a recurring theme, although there have been few major studies of the nature and extent of planning. Ollivant's recollection of his experience is a depressing one: 'The system, however, appeared to take no account of my rights to be consulted or involved in preparations for my future.' He recalls arrangements for boarding out made just before his sixteenth birthday:

'Mr. and Mrs. S came to the Home to meet me a couple of days before I was due to leave. There was no question of asking me whether or not I wanted to leave as all the arrangements had been made. I was given no choice, no consultation and no preparation.'

(Ollivant 1979:72)

This contrasts sharply with the professional prescriptions that are available:

'Preparation for leaving care is crucial. When he leaves, a young person should be at a point in a deliberately planned process. The plan should be in his best interests and should be part of the continuum of planning for him while he has been in care.'

(Mulvey 1977:29)

Finally, in this section some of the key issues are expressed in the following quotations from Godek's (1977) study of twelve adolescents in the months after they left Barnado's Homes:

'For Judy it was the first one to one and a half years after leaving care which presented all the problems for her and it was during this period that she felt the enormous gap between the support she received while in care and then having to find it elsewhere.'

(p. 21)

'(Ann) makes an interesting point about being encouraged to assume independence, but never really being given the power or tools, in a sense, to make decisions independently.'

(p. 18)

'Allan says: "Maybe you could leave for a couple of months to try things out, then maybe you could come back again before you left for good." '

(p. 15)

'Final thought from John who stands 6ft tall: "You feel so small when you leave, the world's a big place!" '

(p. 13)

WHAT ARE INSTITUTIONS FOR?

It has already been suggested here that the reasons for the admission to institutional living will have some influence on the experience of leaving. Goffman's (1961) often-quoted categorization of total institutions provides a useful starting point. He identifies five rough groupings: first, institutions established to care for those who are felt to be both incapable and harmless; second, those for people who are thought to be a threat to the community (albeit unintended) but are incapable of looking after themselves; third, those institutions which are to protect the community from what are regarded as intentional threats; fourth, those established to further some work task; and finally, those designed to serve as retreats from the world. It has often been argued that it is difficult to disentangle the motives of protecting the community from protection of the individual, and it is possible that most admissions to residential care and psychiatric hospitals are based on a combination and a complexity of these motives.

The words in common use to describe the process of leaving give some perspective on this conflict. *Discharge* is a particularly frequent description, but one which is more precisely defined as 'to relieve of load . . . let go . . . put forth . . . get rid of . . . emit' or as 'unloading; firing off of gun; emission (of liquid . . . purulent matter)' (OED). It does, in other words, have rather too many unpleasant associations to be a description of what is also called *release, freedom*, or even *escape*. Perhaps the most extreme expression is the usage of the concept of *disposal*, particularly in medical case conferences in discussion of long-stay patients. Three factors seem to be especially important.

(1) For some people institutional care does represent sanctuary in the sense of escape from intolerable stress in their previous environment. This may range from the child who has been physically attacked by a parent to the prisoner who has been exposed to the strain of the legal process and who may regard prison as the first opportunity to establish a clearly defined and predictable experience for some time (for fuller discussion see Brearley *et al.* (1980)). There is also reason to believe that the similarity and repetitiveness of day-to-day experience in institutions represents a form of security and this predictability may lead to apprehension of change and some difficulty of readjustment for most people who have spent an appreciable time in institutions, whether or not they entered voluntarily.

(2) There are differences between those institutions which are concerned to provide rehabilitation or treatment, those which contain or restrict, and those which are mainly concerned with supporting and providing a safe living environment. The experience of leaving of people admitted against their will must be different from that of people admitted voluntarily and who have found the residential environment enabling and supportive. However, the possibilities for conflict and confusion of aims exists in all cases and it is not enough to assume that all prisoners welcome the end of their sentence without reservation, nor that all young

people are eager to escape to adult life from local authority care. Feelings of abandonment and rejection, of exposure and ambivalence are conspicuous in accounts of leaving, just as much as expressions of feelings of freedom, release, and independence.

(3) It should also be noted that institutional resources are part of a wider organizational context. From the economic viewpoint it is important to make the best use of scarce and expensive institutional resources, to ensure that there is efficient use of the resources to meet a wide and diverse range of needs. In these terms it is perhaps not surprising that in some conditions people begin to be regarded as units to be disposed of in the most efficient manner. An alternative view stresses the social, or humanitarian factors, and begins with the individual perspective. This view emphasizes the importance of initial assessment of the client's need, which must be flexibly and imaginatively matched with what is available to meet that need. Although the focus in this book is on the latter view we are nevertheless very conscious of the importance of economic pressures: we do not and cannot propose an individualized approach which ignores the reality of scarce and inadequate resources.

The view of leaving is likely to be affected by how far losses are anticipated and how these relate to the expected gains, by the extent to which the person feels restrained against his will, and by the degree to which he feels that the purposes of the initial admission have been achieved. In developing this final point some discussion is necessary of the concepts of *outcomes* of institutional living and what has also been called the *outputs* of residential systems.

'Outcomes' is primarily used to refer to the consequences for an individual of the residential experience. Payne (1979), for instance, suggests that in order to understand what can be involved in rehabilitation it is necessary to consider the alternative potential outcomes of a period in care. He distinguishes between primary, secondary, and tertiary rehabilitation. Primary rehabilitation refers to the restoration of a child to the care of his natural parents when this is accomplished as part of a planned and conscious effort by professional workers. Secondary rehabilitation refers to the direction of effort towards successful placement of children in foster care, and tertiary rehabilitation refers to those children who stay in residential care until the statutory leaving age before making their own way in the world. In this sense outcomes refers to the consequences for individuals of a planned series of actions.

A review and discussion of research, policy, and practice in residential homes for the elderly develops the relationship between what are described as the outputs of residential care – 'the quality of life in all its dimensions and other benefits derived from the provision of residential care' – and their determinants, which are called the inputs (Davies and Knapp 1981:5). In these terms outputs include all the consequences which reflect aspects of welfare which are valued in their own right, with particular stress on the importance of a feeling of psychological well-being in the individual. However, the authors also emphasize the enormous complexity of specifying or measuring a clear relationship between inputs and outputs. This is partly because the small scale and enclosed nature of residential settings makes it inevitable that nearly all aspects of the quality of life will be affected by combinations and variations of resources and inputs. It is also noted that variations in inputs do have variable consequences: different people respond differently to similar inputs.

Any discussion of whether residential care, or institutional provision, is in some sense successful must therefore be in the context of the lack of clarity of purpose both in general assumptions about the use of such resources and also often in individual situations. It must also be seen in the light of the difficulty of specifying clear relationships between actions and consequences. There is, however, clear value in a clarification of the concepts of outcome as referring to a relationship between specific planned action with an individual towards expressed goals. Practitioners do operate with assumptions about successful and unsuccessful outcome in these terms. Wills (1970) suggests, for example, that:

'While it is difficult to make even the roughest assessment of outcome, which really cannot be judged for at least five years after discharge, even such judgement as can be made is of little use in assessing the value of a hostel's work unless it is related to our expectations. If those expectations are maintained or exceeded it may be thought that the effort and money have been justified. If expectations are not maintained it may well be thought that the hostel has not justified its existence.'

(p. 123)

In addition to his discussion of success and failure in outcomes Wills also introduces the idea that some departures are premature and this is mirrored in Godek's (1977) question: 'What constitutes maturity or readiness to leave a unit?' (p. 36). Success is likely to be a relative concept and can relate not only to the achievement of the initial goals of admission but also to changing and developing needs, and to planning for the future. The experience of leaving care may be success or failure in relation to previously set objectives, but it may also be successful or unsuccessful in relation to the degree of preparation and disruption which takes place around the actual separation.

As Payne puts it:

'The experience of leaving care has similar components to that of admission. It takes the child from the known to the unknown; from a position of security to one of insecurity. It is accompanied by strong feelings of anxiety, possibly a sense of dread, even of panic at the thought of the prospective changes.'

(Payne 1979:11)

What, then, is the social work role?

SOCIAL WORK AND LEAVING THE INSTITUTION

We will show later how the context of practice and the different needs of client groups influence the actual tasks which the social worker is required to perform. Some elements are, however, common to the process of moving through and out of the institutional system and these will be briefly discussed in order to prepare the basis for a description of positive planning for departure.

(1) Continuity and change

Reference has been made to the importance of leaving care as a major life change. Many will be moving from a familiar to an unfamiliar environment and even those who are returning to a familiar home after a short period in an institutional environment are likely to have experienced important disruptions in their lives. In addition, as many writers have pointed out, valuable relationships with residential staff can be brought to an abrupt end with discharge.

Reactions to loss and change are so much a part of social work practice that it is not necessary to give a detailed repetition here. Probably the most extensively quoted writer on the subject of separation among children has been Bowlby, whose early work (Bowlby 1951) stressed the importance for the child of a continuous relationship with his mother, and this emphasis led to concern about the damaging effect of residential care. More recent findings suggest that long-term negative consequences are likely to be due to a lack of something rather than a loss. Rutter (1972) shows that there is a diversity of effects resulting from various factors which are all grouped under the heading of 'maternal deprivation'. He distinguishes between the disruption of bonding, which probably leads to distress, and the failure of bonding to take place at all, which will be associated with longer-term damage.

The extent to which close relationships with other people in institutions – either staff or residents – develop is very variable and is likely to be related to such things as the length of stay, the previous experience of positive, close relationships, and the extent of unresolved feelings about family relationships, and amongst adults to the extent of intellectual impairment, or of mental illness, etc. It does seem likely that for many people departure will create some loss and therefore at best feelings of distress and unhappiness. Marris (1974) offers a discussion of loss and change which is useful here. He argues that there is a universal impulse to resist change and to retain a meaning in experience which prompts a returning to the past. Loss disrupts our ability to find a continuity of meaning in our experience, and grief represents the struggle to retrieve this sense of meaning 'when circumstances have bewildered or betrayed it' (p. 147). He argues, then, that all change represents loss in so far as it disrupts the familiar meanings which we give to our experiences. To account for the fact that people willingly seek new situations which must inevitably, in his argument, involve them in anxiety, he suggests that 'the innovator accepts the strain of change in order to escape from a more fundamental threat of loss' (p. 2). In these terms, many people seek to leave institutional life (which may create apprehension and fear for the future, as we have seen) because the pains of staying there are even greater: the old lady who resents her loss of independence; the psychiatric patient who fears loss of liberty; the adolescent who seeks growth and maturity; etc.

To extrapolate from this, it is possible to identify ways in which social workers can help to maintain continuity in the lives of clients. Many studies have noted the loss of contact of children in care with their families (Mulvey 1977–78). A period in care for a child will only be a temporary experience, and even if he does not return to his natural parents it is important to retain a sense of identity which involves a knowledge and awareness of the past self (see e.g. Wendelken 1981). On a rather different level it is important to maintain practical continuity of homes and possessions of clients during a period away. This may range from the protection of loved toys for a child to ensuring the safety and maintenance of home and furniture for an elderly, or sick, adult.

It is not only important to maintain this continuity of past and present but also to ensure a continuity of present and future. In many cases this has been achieved by the development of half-way accommodation of various types to help to ease the transition to an open environment. In a discussion of two such ventures for adolescents developed by the Church of England

Children's Society it is suggested that the length of stay in such establishments is crucial, 'with the risk on the one side of inhibiting youth's natural adventurousness by too long a period under supervision and on the other of exposing inadequate young people to situations in which their confidence is bound to be undermined by failure' (Wood 1979). Some not dissimilar issues have arisen in relation to small group homes for those discharged from psychiatric hospital: whether, for instance, they should provide a permanent home for a few individuals, or whether they should provide a final training before more independent accommodation. These practical dilemmas are well illustrated by Rowlett and Dews (1979) in a case example.

Studies have shown the extent of the practical difficulties faced by young people leaving care. Godek (1977) identifies particular problems in the handling of money; the inability of girls (and boys) to cook, sew, and wash clothes for themselves; difficulties in relating with peers and feelings of loneliness; problems of sexuality, particularly in relation to establishing an identity within the peer group; the adolescent dilemma of 'wanting to do things for yourself' but wanting to remain in safety; the difficulties that arise from the ending of long-standing relationships with social work staff; and the development of outside contacts. Although there are practical issues – finding accommodation and employment, handling money, and building up outside relationships – Mulvey (1977–78) suggests that the discharged young adult is not necessarily in a more disadvantaged position than any other young person who leaves home and feels unable to return at times of difficulty. Making a similar point Burgess (1981), in his study of employment and young people leaving residential care, argues that it would be wrong to imply that they are any different from other school leavers, or young people, but comments that 'for most of these youngsters being in care represents just one among many disadvantages' (p. 117).

Practical issues are just as important to other groups of people leaving institutions. A report by NACRO (1980) on work in hostels with single homeless people in Manchester and Stockport, for example, notes that 'some single homeless people display a range of problems including those which require social work skills, others simply need housing. Among both groups homelessness and instability often leads to ill health, continued unemployment and imprisonment for minor offences' (NACRO 1980:1). A study of the need for accommodation for discharged prisoners categorized more than half the men studied as 'quite possibly homeless' (Walmsley 1972). Amongst the elderly, Plank has demonstrated that it is likely to be more costly to discharge people from residential care than to keep them in care, although the differentials depend on the need for services of individual old people (Plank 1977).

The social work role can therefore be concerned with helping to reduce the loss impact of change at the time of departure through contributing to protecting the continuity of life – past, present, and future. Continuity may also be thought of in relation to what has been described as the continuum of care. This concept has been given a number of meanings but in general terms refers to the possibility of using the total range of resources to meet need in the most appropriate way at a point in time. In the prison service context, for example, two quotations illustrate some of the assumptions:

> 'The mode of "through-care" in its ideal form assumes that Probation Officers and Prison Welfare Officers will co-operate closely in providing or offering help from the time of a man's reception into prison until he has re-established himself after release. As in all forms of social work practice, it is no surprise to identify some discrepancy between the ideals and the realities of daily work.'
>
> (Corden *et al.* 1978)

> 'It is suggested that if the question of the homeless prisoner is to be tackled seriously it is necessary to "see things whole". This will entail having a clear means of assessing needs and ensuring that these needs are met. It will also mean seeing the various types of after-care accommodation as part of a system with hostels and lodgings providing a continuum of different degrees and types of support.'
>
> (Walmsley 1972)

In one sense the continuum of service may be seen as a linear experience, with the client entering a system at one end and leaving at the other either undamaged or 'treated', or 'rehabilitated' in some way. As we have already begun to see, and will demonstrate in the following chapters, the institutional experience is not always as positive as this might suggest. Alternatively, the client may be seen as passing through the system with increasing severity of need, receiving different or increased resources to match the need, as, for example, when an old person moves through increasing physical dependency to an ultimate need for long-stay hospital care. The evidence, however, that resources are used interchangeably or as flexibly as the concepts involved here demand is scarce and there is reason to believe that the lack of resources makes such continuity and flexibility unlikely for most people. To take one example, it is well documented that there are some people in old people's homes who would be more appropriately cared for in hospital, and vice versa, but they are unable to move for a number of reasons, not least of which are the administrative and organizational factors. Although some efforts have been made to alter this (see e.g. Braverman and Baldock 1980) the problem remains. Attempts to provide *continuity of service*, in this sense of appropriate allocation of resource to need, may represent a desirable ideal but it is one which has yet to be achieved. It may, of course, not be desirable if there is a greater need for *continuity of experience*: the old person and residential staff may prefer that she should die among familiar faces, even if that involves considerable extra effort, than that she should be moved to hospital for 'better care'.

It is also appropriate to note in this discussion of continuity that moving from one environment to another is potentially stressful and may, as we will show later, actually increase the likelihood of death for frail old people. Any decision about moving people within the caring system − or to the community − should be made with an awareness of this potential stress. It is particularly important to note also that there is evidence that preparation and discussion before the move can help to reduce negative consequences.

(2) Decision-making

The discussion has so far avoided any attempt to distinguish the social work role from that of residential work. To deal with this subject adequately requires much more space than is available here, and the extent of the debate is already considerable. It must be noted however that we will be concerned, in the later discussion, with two distinct kinds of situations. First, there will be discussion of leaving residential settings in which some people are employed as residential workers and have responsibility for domestic as well as social and emotional caring tasks, and sometimes for nursing tasks: in these contexts field social workers from outside the residential unit are involved to a greater or lesser extent in decision-making and in providing certain kinds of help and support to clients. Second, there is consideration of a specific setting – psychiatric hospital – in which the primary tasks of the institutions – custody and treatment – are the responsibility of groups of staff other than social workers: social work in this setting and in some others, such as prisons, is a function performed mainly by a small group of staff based in the institution but employed by agencies outside the institution, and may occasionally also be provided by field social workers from other agencies. The potential for failure of communication, conflict, and other problems in the relationships between social workers and residential workers, care staff and domestic staff, social workers and custodial or medical, field social workers and institution-based social workers, etc. is enormous.

However, the key to positive planning is careful and effective decision-making and considerable attention must be given to these inter-worker issues. The concept of teamwork has been thoroughly considered in recent years and some interesting perceptions have emerged. The predominant view is that effective teamwork is desirable (Lonsdale, Webb and Briggs 1980), although the same authors point out that the assumptions that effective care rests on good teamwork are often based on widely divergent and even conflicting expectations of what can be achieved. In spite of problems in defining types of teams, the overwhelming tendency is to prescribe a team approach. Evers (1981) suggests that the key questions in defining a team include 'Who belongs to the team? What are the team's goals? What is the structure of the team and who is its leader? How does the team make decisions? How is work with patients accomplished by the team, and, most important, what are the care outcomes for patients?' (p. 3). There is an underlying assumption that teams facilitate decision-making and the sharing of knowledge as well as co-operation between team members. Teamwork is not, however, without its problems. In a discussion of case conferences on geriatric patients in hospital, Fairhurst (1977) noted that matters raised related mainly to the work of team members and little reference was made to the patient's perspective. Most time was devoted to discussion of requests for services, profferring of information and reporting back. She comments that conferences are an opportunity for participants to say what work they have done, what this work is, and what it should be. A more detailed study of case conferences about cases of child abuse illustrates the complexity of factors which operate in such situations (Hallett and Stevenson 1980), and it is clear that our knowledge of the processes in team decisions is still very preliminary.

Against this background it remains necessary for different groups of workers to co-operate in order to produce decisions about the future of people in institutions. It might be argued that the most appropriate time to begin to plan for leaving the institution is before admission: the decision to admit should be made in the light of assumptions about goals to be achieved. Certainly it is argued that preparations for departure begin with admission (Payne 1979), and a plan for the total institutional experience should be made. It is more commonly assumed that detailed plans for the future of children in care are appropriate and essential than it is, for example, that similar plans should be made for the elderly, and this perspective is embodied in legislation. However, it will be shown later than this ignores the potential of many older people and we would propose that as a general principle plans for discharge should be considered early in the case of *all* people in institutions.

The relationship between field-work and residential work (and workers) has been thoroughly discussed elsewhere (see e.g. CCETSW 1973; Righton 1973; Slasberg and Godek 1980). Slasberg and Godek suggest that the residential worker is mainly concerned with the position of the resident group as a whole but is as much a vital part of the team as the field-worker. The field-worker, on the other hand, is

> 'mainly responsible for finding another placement, for deciding what type of placement is required, and for the initial work to be done with the client. Although the residential worker may wish to be involved in the work − the statutory responsibility lies with the field-worker and for him/her the whole merry-go-round is beginning once again.'
>
> (p. 13)

The latter point is particularly important in work with children, where the statutory responsibility may continue, but the field social worker's role in following through work with the client after departure is a significant reason for him to be closely involved throughout the process. This does not mean that the residential worker has a lesser role − each has an active and significant part to play.

The involvement of the person most directly affected − the client − is of obvious importance but there is reason to believe that this may not always be encouraged or facilitated. Mention was made earlier, for instance, of the lack of attention to the patient's perspective during geriatric case conferences. Involvement in decision-making will facilitate preparation for, and commitment to the change both in terms of emotional accommodation to the idea of change and in the development of coping skills. Mulvey (1977–78) comments that the tendency to over-protect children in children's homes should not be allowed to prevent them from having the opportunity to shop and budget for themselves. Godek (1977), too, stresses the need for young people to be involved in planning and in preparation for the practicalities of life. Payne argues that 'at all times the child will need to be kept in touch with developments regarding *his* future, not only by involving him in case reviews but through discussion at every available opportunity' (Payne 1979:12). Mulvey summarizes this important aspect clearly: 'Involvement in planning could develop the skill that Parker terms "mastery of the future"' (p. 29). It is also important to recognize the rights of others in decision-making in the life of the resident – particularly those of parents and other family members.

Principle 6 of a BASW Charter of Rights for Children in Care states that 'The child in care has a right to information concerning his circumstances and to participate in the planning of his future' (BASW 1977). It would not be difficult to pursue the importance of the same principle in relation to all groups in institutional care. One positive way towards improving the level of practice and standard of service to clients has been the development of the key-worker concept. In essence the key worker would have responsibility for fulfilling a central role in relation to individual clients. He would be responsible for ensuring that a care plan is evolved; for the implementation of the care plan; for monitoring progress and recommending amendments or changes to the care plan; for calling regular reviews; keeping a working relationship with the client; for maintaining records; and for ensuring arrangements are made for continued social work help where necessary after discharge (RCA/BASW 1978). The decision on which worker would be appointed as the key worker will depend on factors relevant to each individual situation. It represents, therefore, an opportunity to move beyond unproductive debate about generalizations on the respective roles of residential and field-workers to a more individually-focused and flexible perspective.

The purpose of this discussion has been to explore the importance of involvement in decision-making of the various interests and people concerned. It has largely begged the questions which arise from the different contexts of care. It is hardly relevant, for instance, to consider the involvement of a long-term prisoner in a flexible care plan and for many older people the prospect of leaving care after admission is likely to be remote. Nevertheless the basic principle that people have a right to information about their situation and their future and a right to express a view about that future is generally applicable.

Similarly it is important for all people in institutions who have some prospect, however remote, of leaving to be able to plan and prepare for their departure, and for those who will only leave through death it is equally important that there is some conception of an overall purpose to their life and experience. It is, in other words, necessary to plan positively for the continuing experience of all people in institutional situations.

(3) Positive planning

Good planning for leaving the institution begins with careful assessment and planning at the time of admission: appropriate placement and clear and realistic goals in the use of residential care will predispose to a more successful transition at the time of discharge. Principle 3 of the BASW Charter of Rights for Children in Care states that 'Before a child is admitted to care an assessment of his family and home environment should be undertaken which will include the preparation of the child and his family for the admission and their participation in the plans that are made' (BASW 1977 : 7). It can be likewise argued that in relation to the elderly that 'a full assessment is essential following a request for help. This involves subsidiary questions: How much time is there for action? Who wants the action to be taken? How far can the elderly client be involved? What is the relevant information? What are the realistic options?' (Brearley 1976 : 6). The concept of appropriate placement in residential work does, of course, rest on many value assumptions. What follows here, as a statement about the process of entering and leaving institutional situations is intended to be prescriptive. It describes the way we believe that a good or appropriate programme of care should develop in a planned and purposeful way. We recognize that what we suggest does not happen in all cases, and probably not even in most cases, but it represents a desirable approach to strive for. As such it is based on beliefs and values as much as on clear knowledge of a relationship between actions and consequences.

In *Admission to Residential Care* (Brearley *et al.* 1980) we proposed that admission to care is a process moving from the recognition and assessment of hazards or potential danger through a decision on action, preparation and transfer, to arrival and settling in. This process of change through time is similar for a range of settings and types of admission, but it must be recognized that the decisions and approaches made within and in association with the process are affected by various factors and that the time-span and emphases within the process will vary. The following stages are involved in the admission process:

problem perception
investigation and analysis
decision
preparation
transfer
integration
maintenance and recovery

This can now be extended and developed. The experience of living in an institution may also be seen in relation to change over time, and therefore as a process. In an ideal sense, life in care should be concerned with three broad elements: first, with helping the new arrival to settle in, to adapt to the demands of the new environment, and to recover from the distress caused both by the crisis which led to admission and by the actual process of transfer and separation; second, with the provision of an environment which will maintain the level of capacity and abilities of the resident and which may also provide an element of 'holding' or controlling – ranging from provision of consistent authority for the growing child to restraining custody for the long-stay prisoner; third, it should also be concerned with providing scope and opportunities for growth and change. Such a presentation of the institutional process must, however, be set in the context of the purpose of different agencies described earlier. Whilst it may be argued that the primary function of a children's home is to provide a secure, caring environment in which each child can make positive developments, it is much more debatable whether personal growth is a significant component of the hospital task in which the primary function is likely to be focused on the maintenance or restoration of good health. The relative importance of these aspects – integration and repair; holding and maintenance; integrity and growth – will vary amongst different settings and this will be explored in later chapters.

Alongside these issues there is a process which stems from the awareness of the possibility of leaving: the process of departure, which has the following stages:

(a) Planning

As we have already seen this will involve several key elements which will include a *thorough initial assessment*, taking account of the *impact of change* and the central importance of *continuity* of past and present and present and future. It will also involve *making a decision (or decisions)* about the *goals, purposes and objectives* of the placement and about the *implementation* of the plan. This may often involve both short-term and long-term plans ranging from differential diagnosis in the case of an old lady admitted to a hospital geriatric ward for assessment, to a long-term plan for the rehabilitation of a severely handicapped child in care.

(b) Review

It will be necessary to provide a continual check on the implementation of plans to ensure that the placement purposes are being fulfilled. In a discussion of children in care it is suggested that a review should ask the following questions:

'(a) Is the child benefiting from the placement?
'(b) If not why not?
'(c) Can placement amend itself and treatment plan be modified?
'(d) If not, is there a more appropriate alternative?
'(e) If so, is this sufficiently more positive to compensate for the disruption of moving (which is reduced by preparation and follow-up)?'

(Sayer *et al.* 1976:11)

It would seem appropriate to ask similar questions about the experience of adults although, once again, we will consider later the variations which the different settings and contexts may impose.

(c) Preparation

This may be considered in relation to both emotional and practical preparation. Some indication has already been given of the possibilities of helping the individual to retain a concept of continuity in his life and therefore to reduce the impact of change. Godek (1977) highlights three factors which are of particular importance in preparation:

(1) The question of what constitutes maturity or readiness to leave. For some groups – children reaching an appropriate age, prisoners reaching their release date – the question of whether or not they are 'ready' to leave may have little influence on an unavoidable decision. For others, such as hospital patients, some older people, children moving to foster parents or returning to natural parents, etc. this is a very significant question.

(2) The degree of impact that the institution has had on the individual. This may refer to varying issues, from the lack of opportunity for young people to learn about practical tasks such as sewing, cooking and washing to the institutionalizing effect – apathy, withdrawal, ritualized habitual behaviours, etc. – which have been recorded in long-stay psychiatric patients and older people in institutions.

(3) The extent to which the problems which led to the original admission have been dealt with. A depressed, malnourished and confused old lady may recover in hospital but if she is to return to the same lonely, depressing environment a good deal of practical and emotional preparation will be necessary before she can leave.

Good preparation will also include at least two other elements:

(4) The need for practical preparation. This can be considered on two levels: first provision for the material necessities of independent life – accommodation, income, employment,

etc.; and second the acquisition of the skills necessary to independent survival – a young person must learn to operate in the work environment; an ex-psychiatric patient must develop relationships skills; an old person may need to relearn home management skills; etc.

(5) The need to establish supportive relationships which can continue after departure. To quote once more from Godek, who discusses a girl moving from care to a hostel and notes three points:

'(1) The importance of an "outside" person in enabling Ann to look at what was involved in leaving care.

'(2) The initial "facilitating" role of the residential worker in respect of enabling a relationship to grow between Ann and her field-worker.

'(3) The ongoing role of the residential worker after Ann left care.'

(Godek 1977:39)

(d) Departure

The experience of actual separation may be felt in many ways, and perhaps with a sense of anticlimax. It is important for many people that they should not feel that a door is closed completely – that support will be available and that although this may be provided mainly by a field-worker, the residen.ial worker will continue to be available. For others – leaving prison, or hospital, for instance – on one level it will be important that the door *should* be closed: although the need for continuing support will often remain. For many people, as we have shown earlier, ambivalence will predominate: the desire for independence and freedom mixed with the loss of secure and familiar surroundings.

(e) After-Care

Following from this ambivalence it is likely that people will have mixed feelings about support during the period of adjustment or resettlement. One important question for the present discussion concerns the responsibility for the management of this process, and this is closely bound up with the question of where the responsibility of the residential worker or the institution ends. We have drawn attention to the importance of identifying a key worker to take responsibility for ensuring that a plan is made and followed through. If we are to advocate and develop a systematic and purposeful approach to the process of moving into, through, and out of institutional living then this must rest on careful planning. There is, however, some reason to question the effectiveness of intensive post-release or post-discharge involvement (see e.g. Minor and Courlander 1979). It is not possible, therefore, to make specific recommendations about the nature of after-care or about who should provide after-care. Not all people leaving the institutions we discuss here will need or want social work help. For some of those who do need such help it may be best provided by a field-worker, for others continued support from the residential worker will be most appropriate. What is important, however, is a recognition that the process of the residential experience does not finish at departure and a plan for that process should include consideration of after-care needs.

A complete perspective on the process of moving through residential care can therefore be presented (see *Figure 1(1)*).

Finally, it should be stressed that although the process as change through time contains similar elements for all people entering and leaving institutions, the emphases will vary

Figure 1(1)

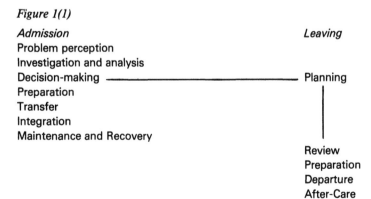

Admission	Leaving
Problem perception	
Investigation and analysis	
Decision-making —————————————	Planning
Preparation	
Transfer	
Integration	
Maintenance and Recovery	
	Review
	Preparation
	Departure
	After-Care

widely, but this overall perspective will be used as a general base for the subsequent discussions, after the detailed description of the most important elements of the legal framework in the next chapter.

2 Legal Aspects
Gwyneth Roberts

Leaving care means transition from life in a protected and/or restricted environment to life in the family and/or the community. It is a process which, in some circumstances, can take place only in accordance with the relevant legal rules. For this reason the legal provisions which govern leaving care can be of considerable significance for the individual concerned as well as for the authority to whose care he has been admitted. In this respect, there is an important distinction to be made between those who have entered care voluntarily and those who came into care as the result of compulsory powers of admission. In principle, the former can leave care at will whenever they choose to do so. The latter, however, can usually leave care only when those powers have been brought to an end, which usually happens in one of two main ways. Authority to detain a person in care can come to an end automatically either when some event occurs or upon the lapse of time; or authority may come to an end through the decision of an individual, such as a doctor, or body, such as a local authority, a court, or a tribunal, which is vested with powers of discharge.

In this chapter, the main legal rules governing leaving care will be discussed in relation to children, the mentally disordered and the elderly. Since powers to detain a person in care are a considerable infringement of an individual's personal freedom, it is important that the law in this respect should be carefully observed so as to avoid either wrongful or unnecessary detention.

CHILDREN

Compulsory powers over children arise in two main ways: when a parental rights resolution is passed in relation to a child in care under Section 2 of the Child Care Act 1980; and when a care order is made in care or criminal proceedings. In both cases compulsory powers over the child vest in the local authority and may last throughout his childhood, unless they are previously brought to an end.

In our society children are usually brought up by their parents within the family unit, and it is generally agreed that this arrangement provides the best environment for a child's physical, emotional, and psychological development. Nevertheless, it is also recognized that in some circumstances it may be necessary in his own interests to separate a child from his parents by admitting him into care. This is a step which can be potentially risky for the child. There is always the danger that he may remain in care simply because no positive action is taken to try to secure his discharge. For this reason, not only do the legal rules set out the relevant procedures through which a child may leave care, but they also place responsibility upon authorities to keep the situation of each child under review and, in some circumstances, to consider whether to apply to the court for his discharge.

Moreover, authorities also have a positive duty to try to secure that a child leaves care if this would be in his interests. Section 1 of the Child Care Act 1980 places a duty upon a local authority to make available such advice, guidance, and assistance as may promote the welfare of children by diminishing the need to keep them in care under the Act. In addition the section gives local authorities power to provide assistance in kind or, in exceptional circumstances, in cash to fulfil this aim. It also enables authorities to call upon other resources in the community to carry out this function since they may make arrangements for the provision of advice, guidance, and assistance by voluntary organizations or by other persons. This Section clearly puts stress upon the importance of supportive case work with families with the aim of reuniting children with their parents.

CHILDREN SUBJECT TO A PARENTAL RIGHTS RESOLUTION

A resolution acquiring parental rights over a child under Section 3 of the Child Care Act 1980 can be passed at any time *if the appropriate grounds exist* in relation to a child already received into care under Section 2 of the Act. A child must be received into care under Section 2 if it appears that he is under seventeen and that he has neither parent nor guardian, or has been or remains abandoned by them, or is lost; or that his parent or guardian are for the time being or permanently prevented by reason of mental or bodily disease or infirmity or other incapacity from providing for his proper accommodation, maintenance, and upbringing, *and* the intervention of the local authority is necessary in the interests of the welfare of the child.

Reception into care can never be against the wishes of a parent, and, in many cases, it comes about as the result of a parental request. The authority acquire no parental rights over the child but must care for him up to the age of eighteen so long as his welfare appears to require it (1980 Act, Section 2(2)). Local authorities also have the duty, *if this would be for his welfare*, to endeavour to secure that a child's care is taken over by a parent or guardian, or by a relative or friend who is of the same religious persuasion, or who undertakes to bring up the child in this religion (Section 2(3)).

There may be circumstances when a parent asks for a child's return but the local authority may feel that it would not be in a child's interests for him to leave care. Since Section 2(3) states that: 'Nothing in this section shall authorise a local authority to keep a child in their care under this section if any parent or guardian desires to take over the care of the child', it might seem that a local social services authority must return the child to a parent or guardian on request. Such a reading of the sub-section might seem in keeping with the principle underlying the voluntary reception of the child in the first place. But it has been held in the *London Borough of Lewisham* v. *Lewisham Juvenile Court Justices [1979] 2 All ER 297* that the power of a local authority to keep a child in their care is not automatically terminated when a parent notifies the authority of his desire to resume care of the child. The authority, however, can then no longer rely upon Section 2 as authorizing them to retain the child, and they must take some other steps to acquire the necessary powers to do so.

If, however, there is a demand by the parents for the immediate return of the child, then it will be difficult in some circumstances for an authority to retain the child long enough to take the necessary steps. If the child has been in care for six months, Section 13 of the 1980 Act is relevant. Under that section, it is an offence to remove a child who has been in the care of the local authority throughout the previous six months unless they consent, or the parent or guardian gives at least twenty-eight days' notice of his intention to take the child out of care. The practical effect of this section, so far as Section 2 is concerned, would seem to be to extend the period of care for twenty-eight days from the date upon which the request for removal was made. During this period, the local authority have time to consider whether they wish to take some further steps to resist the parent's request.

If the child has been in care for less than six months and there is a demand for his immediate return the situation may create problems. According to Lord Salmon, 'once a parent presents herself to the authority and demands the immediate return of the child . . . the child ceases to be in the care of the authority'. Lord Salmon suggested that a local authority might nevertheless consider it to be their moral duty to keep the child long enough to have it made a ward of court, 'although they would have no legal power to do so'. This is perhaps an unfortunate suggestion for social work practice.

In what ways can a local authority acquire further powers over the child while he is in care under Section 2? They may, for example, have grounds for wardship proceedings, but in many cases the action which they will contemplate is the assumption of parental rights.

Passing the resolution

In deciding whether or not to assume parental rights, and so acquire far wider powers over a child, a local authority should have regard to their general duty to him under Section 18(1) of the Child Care Act 1980. Under this section, they have a responsibility in reaching any decision relating to a child in their care to give first consideration to the need to safeguard and promote his welfare throughout his childhood. They must also, as far as is practicable, ascertain the wishes and feelings of the child regarding the decision, and give due consideration to them having regard to his age and understanding.

A resolution assuming parental rights can be passed only on the grounds set out in Section 3 of the 1980 Act. These are (1) that the child's parents are dead and that he has no guardian; or (2) that a parent or guardian (a) has abandoned him; or (b) suffers from some permanent disability rendering him incapable of caring for the child; or (c), while not within (b), suffers from mental disorder within the meaning of the Mental Health Act, 1959 rendering him unfit to have care of the child; or (d) is of such habits or mode of life as to be unfit to have care of the child; or (e) has so consistently failed without reasonable cause to discharge the obligations of a parent as to be unfit to have care of him; or (3) that a resolution is in force in relation to one parent who is, or is likely to become a member of a household comprising the child and his other parent; or (4) that the child has been in the care of an authority under Section 2, or partly in the care of an authority and partly in the care of a voluntary organization for the previous three years.

Through the assumption of parental rights an authority can acquire wide rights and responsibilities over a child initially received into care voluntarily. Section 3 is an exception to the usual rules in that a parent can lose parental rights over a child without that decision being made initially by a court. It can be argued that the grounds set out above are quite specific and that it would be difficult for a parent who is able and willing to provide a satisfactory home environment for a child to lose his rights to his child in consequence of his reception into care. But the grounds which allow a local authority to acquire parental rights over a child because he has been in care for three years have been subject to criticism. The duty to work toward the rehabilitation of a child to his parents should always be borne in mind by local authorities in relation to a child in their care.

Any person deprived of his parental rights in this way, and

who has not consented to the resolution, must be given notice of the fact if his whereabouts are known. He may then serve a written counter-notice on the authority objecting to the resolution. The resolution will then lapse automatically unless within fourteen days of the counter-notice being served the authority apply to a juvenile court for an order that the resolution should not lapse. The resolution remains in force during this period. In order to secure the continuance of the resolution the authority must satisfy the court (1) that the ground upon which the resolution was originally passed was made out, (2) that there continue to be grounds (perhaps not the original ones) on which a resolution can now be founded, and that it is in the interests of the child (Section 3(6)).

If the resolution is not upheld by the court it will lapse and the child may be removed. The authority can, however, appeal to the High Court against the refusal of the court to confirm the resolution. A parent, too, may appeal if the resolution is upheld.

If it is upheld the resolution remains in force either until the child is eighteen or until it is brought to an end by the authority or by a court. The authority itself can rescind the resolution at any time if that appears to be for the child's benefit (Section 5(3)) or a parent who has been deprived of his rights may apply to the juvenile court within six months of the resolution alleging that there were no grounds for passing the resolution (Child Care Act 1980, Section 5(4); Magistrates' Courts Act 1952, Section 127(1)). He may also apply to court at any time on the grounds that the resolution should be terminated in the child's interests (1980 Act, Section 5(4)). The burden of proof on these two occasions is on the parent so that his task is more difficult than it is under the objection procedure. There is again a right of appeal to the High Court both against an order bringing the resolution to an end, and against a refusal to do so. It is not clear what weight should be given to 'the benefit of the child' or to 'the interests of the child' under these sections.

The resolution will also be brought to an end if the child is adopted, or if a guardian is appointed under Section 5 of the Guardianship of Minors Act 1971 (Child Care Act 1980, Section 5(2)).

Parental rights resolutions can be passed to deprive only one of the parents of the child of his rights in relation to the child (1980 Act, Section 3(1)). In this case the parent who retains his rights will share them with the authority. It is unlikely, however, that he could discharge the child from care. A putative father is not a 'parent' for the purposes of the Child Care Act 1980, and so he has no parental rights in relation to the child. If he wishes to obtain custody he can apply to the court under the Guardianship of Minors Act 1971, when the test to be applied will be the welfare of the child.

CHILDREN IN CARE UNDER A CARE ORDER

The second main way in which a local authority become vested with compulsory powers over a child is through a care order made either in care proceedings brought under Section 1 of the Children and Young Persons Act 1969, or in criminal proceedings where the child has been found guilty of an offence which would be punishable with imprisonment in an adult (1969 Act, Section 1(1) and Section 7(7)(a)).

The general duty of a juvenile court in dealing with a child brought before it in any proceedings is to have regard for his welfare and, in appropriate cases, to take steps to remove him from undesirable surroundings and secure that proper provision is made for his education and training (Children and Young Persons Act 1933, Section 44).

Care proceedings under Section 1 must be based on one or more of the seven specific grounds set out in Section 1(2) and the court must also be satisfied that the child is in need of care and control which he is unlikely to receive unless an order is made. The seven grounds are:

(1) that the child's proper development is being avoidably prevented or neglected or his health is being avoidably neglected or he is being ill-treated;

(2) that it is probable that condition (1) will be satisfied having regard to the fact that the court or another court has found the condition satisfied in the case of any other child who is or was a member of the household to which he belongs;

(3)   that it is probable that condition (1) will be satisfied having regard to the fact that a person who has been convicted of an offence mentioned in Schedule 1 of the 1933 Act is or may become a member of the same household as the child;

(4)   that he is exposed to moral danger;

(5)   that he is beyond the control of his parents;

(6)   that he is of compulsory school age and is not receiving full-time education suitable to his age, ability, and aptitude;

(7)   that he is guilty of an offence (excluding homicide).

Although condition (7) allows care proceedings in relation to a child of ten years of age or over to be based upon the allegation of an offence (excluding homicide) this procedure is rarely used since it is easier simply to prosecute the child when it is not necessary to show that the child is in need of care and control.

If at the end of *care* proceedings a court is not in a position to decide what final order to make, it is possible for it to make an interim care order which commits the child into the care of the local authority for any period of time up to the maximum of twenty-eight days (1969 Act, Section 2(4), 20 (1)). Before the expiration of an interim care order, either the child or the authority may apply to the juvenile court for it to be discharged under Section 21(2) of the 1969 Act. The child may also apply to the High Court for discharge under Section 22(4) of the Act, but if he is unsuccessful then he cannot be allowed to live at home without the court's consent. If the order is not discharged, then the child must be brought before the court at or before the expiry of the interim care order when the court may again make an interim care order although it will usually come to a final decision. A child may also be remanded in custody or on bail before or during *criminal* proceedings. If he is refused bail then he will normally be committed into the care of a local authority (1969 Act, Section 23(1)) for a period not exceeding twenty-one days (Magistrates' Courts Act 1980, Section 10(2)).

If a care order is made at the end of care or criminal proceedings then it is the duty of the local authority 'to receive the child into their care, and, *notwithstanding any claim by his parent or guardian*, to keep him in their care while the order . . . is in force' (1980 Act, Section 10(1)). The authority have no power themselves to release the child from care. This situation is different in this respect from that which exists when a resolution under Section 3 of the 1980 Act has been passed. The only competent authority which can bring *care orders* to an end is a court.

What are the procedures for doing so? There is a system of appeal against conviction and sentence in all criminal proceedings, and a child also has a right of appeal against the making of a care order under Section 1 of the 1969 Act (1969 Act, Section 2(12)).

If an appeal fails and the child remains in care, then the care order can be discharged by the court at any time on the application of the authority, or of the child (1969 Act, Section 21(2)), or of his parents on his behalf (1969 Act, Section 70(1)). In deciding whether or not to apply to the court for the discharge of a care order, the authority should be governed by the provisions of Section 18(1) of the Child Care Act 1980 discussed above (see page 38). However, they should also bear in mind their duties under Section 18(3) and under Section 19 of the 1980 Act which, in order to protect members of the public, can override their duty under Section 18(1). Consideration of the need to apply to the court arises in particular in the course of six-monthly reviews which an authority must conduct in relation to each child in care under whatever statutory provision. If the child is subject to a care order, then the authority must also consider in his case whether or not to apply for its discharge (1969 Act, Section 27(4)).

The grounds upon which a care order can be discharged are that the court considers that it would be appropriate to do so. If the child is under eighteen, a supervision order may be made. If, however, he appears to be in need of care or control, the court must not make an order unless it is satisfied that he will receive that care and control either through the making of a supervision order or otherwise (1969 Act, Section 21(2)). It is the applicant, whether local authority or child, who must satisfy the court that the child will receive the care and control which he needs if the order is discharged. The court must also, in reaching its decision, have regard to its duty under Section 44 of the 1933 Act (p. 41).

It has been suggested that in the discharge of a care order, 'the way in which "appropriate" and "care and control" are defined is clearly of crucial importance', and that in practice 'appropriate' is often defined 'in terms of the "fitness" of the parents and the quality of care and control they can currently provide' (Adcock and White 1980:259). The authors suggest that the extent to which the court has regard to the welfare of the child will be a matter of individual choice. They contrast this with the position of the court where it is required to reach a decision on an application to rescind a Section 3 resolution where it is clearly required to decide in the interests of the child and the onus is on the parent to show that this is so. Adcock and White are particularly concerned with the effect this may have in the case of deprived or abused children. They argue that the question of parental fitness in these cases should be made subordinate to the needs of the child.

If an application for the discharge of a care order is *unopposed* then the court must order that a parent should not be treated as representing the child or acting on his behalf (unless the court is satisfied that to do so is unnecessary to safeguard his interests). The court must then appoint a guardian *ad litem* for the child unless it is satisfied that to do so is unnecessary to safeguard his interests. By this means, an attempt is made to consider the welfare of the child apart from the interests of either the local social services authority or the child's parents.

If an application for the discharge of a care order is refused then no further application can be made within three months without the consent of the court. However, an appeal against refusal to discharge a care order lies to the Crown Court.

If an order has not been discharged during his childhood the child will automatically leave care when he reaches the age of eighteen, unless he was sixteen when the order was made, in which case it lasts until he is nineteen (Section 20(3)), or unless the authority applies for its extension to the age of nineteen under the terms of Section 21(1).

In this section, the main legal provisions which govern discharge of children from care have been outlined. The discussion has not, however, been exhaustive, and social workers should be aware of the possible relevance of other procedures, such as wardship, guardianship, or adoption in bringing local authority care to an end. The possible interest of individuals other than the authority, the parents, or the child in decisions relating to discharge from care should also be borne in mind. The position of foster parents is particularly relevant in this respect. Readers are referred to the literature mentioned later in this chapter in which these issues are discussed.

THE MENTALLY DISORDERED*

Social and legislative policy towards the mentally disordered attempts to strike a balance between the freedom which an adult normally enjoys and the need to protect him in those circumstances where he is regarded as vulnerable or dangerous because of his mental state. Whether the balance which is now being struck is in the best interests of the mentally disordered is the subject of much current concern and debate. The question is one which closely affects the 20,000 or so who are admitted into a psychiatric hospital in any year.

> 'Detention in such an institution deprives them of the company of their families and friends, of opportunities to pursue their careers and other interests, and of a vast range of activities which the rest of us take for granted. All these deprivations are the direct consequence of the fact that compulsory detention in a psychiatric institution involves the loss of liberty.'
>
> (Gostin and Rassaby 1981:xviii)

The policy behind the Mental Health Act 1959 is that the treatment of the mentally disordered should as far as is possible be based on informal admission into hospital. Indeed, almost 90 per cent of patients suffering from mental illness or handicap are in hospital voluntarily and 95 per cent of residents at any

---

* The section on the mentally disordered was prepared before the Mental Health (Amendment) Bill was introduced. This discussion is based on proposals for reform contained in the White Paper, *Review of the Mental Health Act* (DHSS 1978b).

one time are in this category (DHSS 1978b). What is the legal status of these patients? Do they, for example, have the same rights to leave hospital as patients who are undergoing care and treatment because of a physical disease? Informal patients, like patients who are physically ill, can discharge themselves at any time. There is, however, the possibility of being detained for up to three days while an application for compulsory admission is made if the doctor in charge of the patient's treatment thinks that that is necessary, and also that the grounds for compulsory admission exist. The Review of the Mental Health Act (DHSS 1978b) suggests that since Section 30 could be applied to any hospital patient who becomes mentally disordered, it cannot be said to differentiate informal psychiatric patients from others. This, however, is akin to special pleading. It can hardly be said that the possibility of Section 30 being used in relation to them will be an appropriate consideration in the minds of non-psychiatric patients, whereas its very existence may seem to psychiatric patients to contain an implied threat that compulsory measures may be taken to detain them if they refuse the treatment offered. Current government proposals to amend the Act do not propose modifying the substance of Section 30. On the contrary, it is proposed to extend the scope of the Section to give a registered mental nurse a 'holding power' of up to six hours to enable a report to be obtained from either the doctor in charge of the patient's treatment or his nominated deputy. This proposal meets the complaint which has been made by hospital staff that the doctor in charge of the patient's treatment is not always immediately available. This proposal has been criticized on the grounds that it might have been thought that the 'overall aim would be to reduce powers as much as possible not extend them to new occupational groups' (Bean 1979:105).

The White Paper proposes that all informal patients should be given a written statement of their rights, including the right to leave hospital if they wish. Where a patient's status is changed, it is proposed that the patient should be informed in writing within twenty-four hours of the change in status and of the conditions and rights appropriate to his new status. These proposals will, it is hoped, help informal patients who 'rightly or wrongly, feel themselves to be under a degree of coercion. Others, while not detained under the Mental Health Act, may, because of their mental state, be unable to assert a wish to leave hospital or to refuse consent to a particular form of treatment. There have also been occasions when it has not been made clear to patients that they have ceased to be subject to compulsory powers and thus as informal patients they are free to leave hospital if they wish.'

(DHSS 1978b : 4)

DISCHARGE OF DETAINED PATIENTS

There are two main ways in which compulsory powers come into existence in relation to the mentally disordered: either as the result of an application for admission under Part IV of the Mental Health Act 1959, or as the result of a hospital order made under Section 60 of the 1959 Act. In both cases, the power of compulsory detention will in general come to an end automatically after the maximum period for detention has passed. There are, however, exceptions to this rule which will be discussed below. Detention may also be brought to an end by the action of a person or body which has the necessary authority to discharge the patient. The function and role of the Mental Health Review Tribunal is particularly important in this respect.

Lapse of time

An application for compulsory admission into hospital made under some sections of the 1959 Act involves detention for a relatively short time. Admission for observation under Section 25 provides for detention for up to twenty-eight days. It cannot be renewed and any further detention can only be on the basis of an application for admission for treatment. The White Paper proposes that this should be made clear in the legislation. Section 29 provides for the removal of a patient to hospital for observation in an emergency for up to seventy-two hours on the recommendation of one medical practitioner. The period may be extended, however, if a second medical recommendation is given as required by Section 25 for admission for observation.

An application for long-term admission for treatment can be made under Section 26 of the Act. Detention under this Section is for one year in the first instance but it can then be renewed for a further year and for subsequent periods of two years. The White Paper proposes that the period of detention should be halved to six months, followed by a further six months, and then for one year at a time.

Hospital orders can be made under Section 60 of the Act if a person convicted in the magistrates' court or in the Crown Court is considered to be suffering from mental disorder which warrants detention in hospital and the court considers that, having regard to all the circumstances, this is the most suitable method for disposing with the case. In effect admission to hospital is on a similar basis to that of a patient admitted for treatment under Section 26, and the same time limits will apply. If, however, the Crown Court is also satisfied that the protection of the public requires it, having regard to the nature of the offence, the antecedents of the offender and the risk of his committing further offences if set at large, the court may make the order under Section 65 with restrictions on discharge. A magistrates' court may remit an offender to the Crown Court for an order to be made. The patient can then only be discharged with the consent of the Home Secretary. There is, however, the possibility of appealing against the making of the order.

Apart from these maximum periods (subject to extension in some cases) for which patients may be detained, they may also cease to be subject to powers of detention if they stay away from hospital with or without leave of absence.

Leave of absence may be given by the responsible medical officer (RMO) either indefinitely or for a specified period. If a patient has been continuously on leave for six months then he cannot be recalled to hospital unless at the end of his period of leave he is absent without leave. This does not apply if the patient is on a restricted hospital order since he can then be recalled by the Home Secretary at any time. It is proposed that if a restricted patient is recalled, the matter should be referred to a tribunal within a month of recall (DHSS 1978).

Absence without leave can also result in discharge from care. If a patient detained under Section 26 or Section 60 is not recaptured during twenty-eight days of continuous absence then he is no longer liable to detention (unless subject to a restriction order). The White Paper proposes that no time limit should apply to short-term powers of detention, that is Sections 29, 25, and 30.

Discharge by the decision of a competent authority

The RMO or the hospital managers can discharge a compulsory patient (except a restricted patient) at any time when he is in hospital, and even before the expiration of his maximum period of detention (Section 47(3)). Their powers in this respect are total and may be exercised even if the grounds upon which the patient was originally detained exist.

The nearest relative (defined in Section 49 of the Act) may discharge a patient who is subject to detention under Section 26 (but not Section 60) of the Act by giving seventy-two hours' notice in writing. The RMO may then provide the hospital managers with a report certifying that in his opinion the patient would, if discharged, be likely to act in a manner dangerous to himself or to others. This bars the nearest relative from himself discharging the patient for six months, although he may apply within twenty-eight days to a Mental Health Review Tribunal. The nearest relative may also be barred by an application being made to the county court for his removal if he exercises his powers of discharge, or is likely to do so, without having due regard to the welfare of the patient or the interests of the public (1959 Act, Section 52(3)(d)).

It is the Home Secretary alone who can discharge a patient who is subject to a hospital order with restriction under Section 66. If he discharges the patient then he may either grant an absolute discharge or he may attach conditions that the patient is subject to compulsory after-care and re-call to hospital. Discharge can take place at any time but it is usually granted only after the RMO has recommended that course. The Home Secretary must then consider if, in the circumstances of the case, there would be a risk to the public were the patient to be discharged. If so, he will refer the matter for consideration to the Advisory Board on Restricted Patients.

The main safeguard for patients in hospital under compulsory powers, however, is the Mental Health Review Tribunal set up under the 1959 Act with the function of acting as an independent body to consider applications for discharge. Each tribunal consists of a legally qualified president, a doctor, and a lay person. The medical member examines the patient and his records before the hearing. Mental Health Review Tribunals have been subject to a number of criticisms in recent years, some of which will be considered here.

One criticism of the current rules is that short-term patients are barred from applying to a Mental Health Review Tribunal. At present a patient in hospital under Section 26 can apply within six months of admission or within six months of reaching the age of sixteen, whichever of these is the later, and once in each period of renewal of detention (Sections 31(4)(5), 41(5), 43(6), and 63(4)). A patient admitted to hospital under Section 60 may also apply to the tribunal as if he was detained under Section 26. A patient aged sixteen who has been re-classified can apply within twenty-eight days of being informed of the fact. But patients who are admitted for observation or who are in hospital under a restricted hospital order have no right to go to the tribunal under the provisions of the 1959 Act.

The patient's nearest relative may apply to a tribunal within twenty-eight days of receiving the notice that he has been barred from discharging the patient by the issue of a report by the RMO. He may also apply within twenty-eight days of being notified of the patient's re-classification. A nearest relative can also apply once every twelve months when he has been deprived of his powers to act by the County Court, and once every twelve months in relation to a patient held under a hospital order without restriction.

A patient subject to a restriction order can ask the Home Secretary to refer his case to a tribunal in his second year of detention and then once in every subsequent two-year period. The Home Secretary must refer the case to the tribunal within two months of receiving the request but is not bound by the tribunal's recommendation. He may also refer a case to a tribunal himself for advice at any time.

The White Paper considered the current legal rules governing entitlement and recommended that they should be changed in line with their other proposals for reducing the periods for which patients could be detained. This would mean that a patient detained under Sections 26 or 60 (without restrictions) could refer his case to a tribunal during the six-month period for which he was detained, followed by once in the subsequent six months and once within the subsequent year. Restricted patients would have no access to a tribunal during the first year of detention but would be entitled to be referred once during the second year and then annually.

These changes would meet some of the criticism which has been voiced over the current position of detained patients. In themselves, however, they do not meet the problem of the patient who lacks initiative to apply. The White Paper, therefore, proposes automatic reviews by tribunals of patients who have not availed themselves of their right to apply. The reviews would be held after six months for unrestricted patients, then within three years of admission, and thereafter at three-yearly intervals. The interval could possibily be reduced by regulations in the light of experience. For restricted patients, automatic reviews would take place at three-yearly intervals of those patients who had not exercised their right to request referral within the preceding three years.

Another area of concern which is discussed in the Review Document is that of the tribunal's powers. These are currently restricted to either discharging the patient immediately or to re-classifying him as suffering from another mental disorder. Section 123(1) of the Act allows them to direct that an un-restricted patient should be discharged on any grounds but it *must* order discharge in some circumstances. The new proposals would enable tribunals also to order delayed discharge for up to three months: to recommend trial leave. or transfer to another hospital, or conditional discharge. When a recommendation was made it would take into account the need for agreement with other authorities so that tribunals would be able to make an alternative finding if their recommendations could not be implemented.

The White Paper also proposes that an application should not be withdrawn without the tribunal's consent, and that, if withdrawn before being heard, that should not prevent a further application being made within the specified period. These proposals would meet the concern felt by MIND that pressure is sometimes placed upon patients to withdraw an application, by, for example, the promise of imminent discharge, and also meets the difficulty that a patient has the right to make only one application in a specified period.

Tribunal membership is also discussed. It is suggested that greater use should be made of members with social services experience and that a fourth member of the tribunal should be appointed where appropriate. Membership might include social workers with experience in the field of mental health or psychiatric nurses. It is also proposed to involve forensic psychiatrists more frequently in tribunal work.

MIND feels that the reforms set out in the White Paper and other recent government publications promise a basis for improvement in the operation of the Mental Health Review Tribunals. Nevertheless, it feels that 'more far-reaching changes are required if adequate provision is to be provided for the liberty of detained patients' (Gostin and Rassaby 1980:157).

THE ELDERLY

Most elderly people enter care without the use of compulsory powers. The one statutory provision which allows for their compulsory admission is Section 47 of the National Assistance Act 1948 as amended by the National Assistance (Amendment) Act 1951.

Section 47 aims at securing care and attention for any person who

(1) suffers from grave chronic disease or who, being aged, infirm, or physically incapacitated, is living in insanitary conditions, and

(2) is unable to devote to himself, and is not receiving from other persons, proper care and attention.

Action is initiated by a community physician who, after a thorough inquiry, certifies in writing to a district council or a London Borough Council or the Common Council of the City of London that, in the person's own interests, or to prevent injury to the health of, or serious nuisance to other persons, it is necessary to remove him from the place where he is living.

The authority may then apply to the local magistrates' court after giving seven clear days' notice to the person to be removed, or to the person in charge of him, of the time and place of the application. No order can be made unless the manager of the premises to which it is proposed to remove the person concerned has also been given seven days' notice of the time and place of the intended application, except where the manager himself attends the hearing and is heard by the court.

If the court is satisfied by evidence given orally in the court to support the written allegations, it may, if it considers that to be expedient, order the person's removal for any period up to three months. The order can thereafter be renewed indefinitely.

A person who has been compulsorily removed under a Section 47 order may apply for its revocation at any time after six clear weeks from when it was made. He, or the person making the application on his behalf, must also give the community physician seven days' notice of the time and place of the hearing. The court may then revoke the order if in the circumstances it appears expedient to do so.

In some circumstances it is possible to remove a person without giving him notice. In this case the community physician and another doctor must, after a thorough inquiry, consider it necessary in the interests of the person to remove him without delay. In this case the application can be made either to a local magistrates' court or to a single justice. If the manager of the premises has agreed to receive the person to be removed, he need not either be heard by the court or alternatively be given notice of the application. The order can, if the court or justice thinks it necessary, be made *ex parte*, that is, without the person himself, or a representative taking part in the proceedings. Orders made under this procedure can last up to three weeks and cannot be revoked (National Assistance (Amendment) Act 1951, Section 1(3)).

There is little information available about the use made of these procedures for compulsory removal. One survey of the use of Section 47 was carried out in 1979 by means of a questionnaire sent to all community physicians responsible for the Section and 90.8 per cent of the sample responded. Their answers showed that, on average, 207 people were removed annually between 1974 and 1978, of which 94 per cent were removed using 1951 Act powers (Gray 1980a). He suggests that Section 47 should be amended so that social workers are always involved in cases where compulsory removal is being considered.

SUMMARY

In this chapter some of the main pathways out of compulsory care have been considered, and some of the weaknesses in the current situation have been outlined. For further discussion readers are also referred to the following: Hoggett (1976) and (1981); McClean (1980); Roberts (1981). This is an area of the law which has perhaps been somewhat neglected by social workers and lawyers in the past. There is, however, a growing body of informed opinion which is concerned with strengthening the rights of those in care not only by reform of the actual procedures for bringing detention to an end but also by ensuring that information and advocacy in this area are more readily available. Legal safeguards which are little used are of little value. The questions raised here, as in the chapter on admission into care (Brearley *et al.* 1980), highlight once more the tension which inevitably exists between the concept of freedom of the individual on the one hand, and the concept of welfare and protection on the other. Whether a proper balance between the two is always achieved in this area of the law should be a matter of concern to social workers, who, by the nature of their functions and role, are so closely involved in these issues.

Part Two

Introduction   *Paul Brearley*

As we have already suggested, the first three chapters of this section focus on the needs of children and of older adults, since work in institutional situations with these groups is more easily recognizable in the term 'residential work'. This does present a number of difficulties, not least of which is the fact that many children with handicaps are likely to spend some time in hospitals as well as in residential homes. Similarly, older people are likely to move between hospital and residential homes, and many of the arguments which we apply to the experience of leaving are equally relevant to each situation. Although we have tried to deal with the different implications where they exist, we have assumed, in Chapters 4 and 5, that the principles of good practice which we discuss are equally applicable to hospitals and homes and we have avoided clumsy repetition of this proposition as far as possible.

Also in an attempt to avoid duplication, the two chapters which are concerned with the needs of children have each developed a very different approach. In Chapter 3 attention is given to the emotional needs of children, in whatever setting, and to the responsibility of workers, whatever their role, to provide for the need of individual children to receive trusting, caring, and honest relationships which will support their growth and development, not only in the residential home but as a basis for the years to follow. This theme is also maintained in the following chapter, which is concerned with children with handicaps, but here attention is drawn much more to the total resource context within which care can be provided for such children. To some extent the decision to slant the chapters in these ways was inevitable — it is much easier to give attention to social work during the process of leaving care for children in general for a number of reasons, but particularly because there is a more extensive literature and a common assumption in practice that social workers (both field and residential) should and will be involved with children throughout their experience in residential care. In the case of handicapped children, however, the policy issues are much less clear and although there seems to be general acceptance in principle that they should receive the same kind of care and level of social work support, there does seem to be reason to question the lack of clarity in policy and practice with this group.

A further issue of potential duplication in this section lies in the respective roles of the professionals involved. Each chapter draws attention to different aspects of this. In Chapter 3 general prescriptions are made for the role of the social worker, who is referred to as 'key worker'. In practice this may be the residential worker or a field social worker, or even, at different times, both of these, and, as we have argued in the first chapter, the decision on which worker is the most appropriate will depend on a wide range of factors – the client, the workers, the extent of previous involvement, the stage of the process, the action proposed, etc. We do not wish to repeat this argument here in detail and for the present purposes the important points to note are that the broad principles laid down should provide a basis for practice, whoever the worker, and – perhaps most important of all – that a decision must be made about the detailed responsibilities of all the workers involved. A rather different aspect of this is brought out in Chapter 4 in the recognition of the respective responsibilities of different professional groupings who are likely to become involved at times of transition and throughout the residential experience of some people. This is also a feature of the discussion of older people in Chapter 5 where attention is particularly drawn to the importance of shared decision-making involving the client and his family as well as the workers.

There has been considerable discussion of the nature of the social work task in residential care. Ward (1980) suggests that,

'Social work in a residential setting is about working with people in a shared day-to-day living experience. Whether the task is providing care for the aged in an old people's home, or containing critically damaged boys and girls inside a locked unit, it is what is going on between the people involved that determines the quality of residential care.'

(p. 25)

Whilst it is generally found reasonable to acknowledge the central importance of interactions and relationships between people in residential care, there are considerable difficulties in identifying the boundaries between those kinds of institutional living which can be described as residential care and other forms of institutional life. There is, for instance, a shared day-to-day living experience in hospitals and prisons, but these have not usually been described in the same terms as residential care.

In the final chapter of this section there is discussion of some of the issues arising in relation to social work in psychiatric hospitals, in which the predominant purpose relates to issues such as treatment and containment, with the provision of food, warmth, and other facilities to maintain the basic necessities of life taking a secondary, if essential place. It is, of course, important in any institution that these basic needs are efficiently met in order that the primary task of the institution is facilitated: treatment, rehabilitation, therapy, containment, control, etc. In the residential care situation, however, the *process* by which primary needs are met is also an important aspect of meeting the purpose of the establishment: caring for people, in other words, provides the basis of the helping.

In Chapter 6 the discussion of psychiatric hospitals puts considerable stress on the potentialities of the social work contribution to a multi-disciplinary context. It is too simplistic to suggest that social work is a subsidiary function in hospitals, and medicine or psychiatry the primary function. The relationship between professional inputs is complex and social workers can make a significant contribution to the experience of many psychiatric patients – not least in relation to the continuity of that experience and after-care. Particularly important in this setting is the potential for conflict between the aims, values, and effects (both formal and informal) of the institutional system and the expressed objectives and values of social work.

Although it is inappropriate to describe departure from hospital as 'leaving residential care' we believe that the four chapters in this section amply demonstrate that there are common elements in the transitional process. It is important to learn the lessons from each context and thereby broaden our understanding of similar situations. In summary, we have tried to illustrate a variety of perspectives by giving each chapter a different general orientation, whilst still maintaining the central theme of leaving care as a process. We believe that several different strands for action emerge. There is clearly a role for the planner and policy-maker in the need to establish overall approaches which recognize the importance of creating a range of different opportunities and services. There is, similarly, a management role in the deployment of available resources in the most imaginative ways possible. Finally, there are prescriptions for the practitioner who must operate within a restricted set of services with limited resources but who must still find ways of helping individuals both to grow and to lead a successful, satisified life within residential environments and to find ways out from them.

In practice it is probably the residential worker who will have the primary role in carrying out the plan for each person in care, and therefore in preparing for departure, in spite of the fact that the statutory duty, and often the responsibility for decision-making, may be imposed on the field-worker. What is important is that the work does not fall on any one worker by default: it should be the result of a planned and agreed decision made at the beginning of a placement in residential care and subject to regular review. This discussion is not aimed at either residential workers or field-workers in particular. We believe that either could appropriately carry out most of the tasks that will be outlined, but we also recognize the potential conflict and confusion which can arise and which must be guarded against, and that these comments must be viewed in relation to the special opportunities which living and working alongside people on a day-to-day basis can create.

3 Children *Penny Gutridge*

The subject of children leaving residential care brings to mind those young people who are about to attain adult status and for whom no statutory responsibility remains after their eighteenth birthday. A moment's reflection however brings the realization that children may leave residential care at any age, for a number of different reasons, and for a variety of possible destinations.

Children who leave residential establishments and residential social workers to live elsewhere with other people may range in age from very young to school leaving age and beyond; they may have been in residence for lengths of time varying from a few days or weeks to several years; they may have lived in more than one residential setting in more than one locality; they may be alone and without siblings, or placed with a sibling(s), or have siblings dispersed elsewhere; they may or may not know of, or maintain contact with, a parent(s) or relative(s); they may have had a relatively uncomplicated passage, enjoying constant care and attention, actively involved in life inside and outside the institution and consciously engaged with trusted adults in planning and preparing for their futures; or, as seems more likely, they may have had a chequered history of pass the parcel experiences, broken relationships and promises, with little or no sense of control over events and associated feelings, culminating in low self-esteem and self-confidence, little trust in self or others, and minimal hope for the future.

It is these latter children who will be gravely at risk; in danger of becoming those hollow individuals described by Fraiberg (1959) – isolated, detached, emotionally sterile, and unable to give what they have never received and learned from personal experience. Averting this outcome for children will be of as much concern here as it was in relation to admission to residential care (Gutridge 1980).

The point has been made already that the experience of leaving residential care cannot be divorced from that of admission; from the reasons for admission; the extent to which purposes have been realized, objectives met, and goals achieved; from the gains made during residence and the losses endured before and since admission. Attention has been drawn to the fact that outcomes of admission, residence, and leaving residential care should be the consequences of a planned series of actions, a matter of design and not accident, and that one significant result, or output, of a period in residence should be a sense of well-being; a realistic optimism born of a confidence and competence appropriate to the new situation and arising from the quality of input, or care received and social work practised, in the residential setting left behind.

Outcomes for children vary. Acknowledging Payne's distinction between primary, secondary, and tertiary rehabilitation (1979) it is clear that, as a consequence of a planned series of actions, children may return to a parent(s) or relative(s), or begin anew with substitute parents – foster or adoptive – or they may reach statutory leaving age and have to make their own way in the world. Alternatively they may move to another residential establishment for reasons associated with their social, emotional, educational, or health needs, or because of changed circumstances in their family of origin, or even for reasons to do with agency expediency such as home closure in response to financial constraints. Young people may transfer to quite different institutions such as hospitals, or hostels, or the armed forces to train and work; there are times when children make their own spontaneous decisions and run away, and there are other times when the ultimate decision is beyond anyone's control and a child who is terminally ill, or fatally injured, dies whilst in residential care. These last two groups demand their own particular kind of attention from social work staff. Care of a child facing death, and of significant other people associated with the child and likely to be deeply affected, raises issues beyond the scope of this chapter (Anthony 1973; Burton 1974; Lonsdale, Elfer, and Ballard 1979) but some consideration will be given to runaway children.

For some reason departure – its precursors and postscripts – has been a neglected area of study. Parker (1980) points out that although in most years nearly as many children pass out of public care as enter, the point of departure has attracted comparatively little attention (1980). The authors refer to cessation of statutory responsibility for children 'in the care of the council' in the broadest sense but amongst those passing out of public care annually will be a proportion of children leaving residential care. Add to their number those leaving voluntary residential care whose costs are not paid from public funds and one wonders why it is that departures from residential care in particular have not provoked more interest and analysis given the intimacy of group living and the presumed significance of the event for children and care-takers alike.

Where attention has been drawn to leaving residential care it had tended to focus upon children about to become adults, and upon feelings and expectations experienced by young people either in anticipation or in retrospect. Little seems to be known about younger children's thoughts on the matter although there is some related material (see e.g. Tizard 1977) but personal witness to the stress evoked at the prospect of leaving residential care in adolescence stretches across decades to the present generation (Hitchman 1966; Thomas 1967; Page and Clark 1977; O'Neill 1981) making one yet more curious about why there has been so little consideration of the subject in print by those with professional concern and responsibility. For what literature there is on the subject we are indebted to progressive voluntary child care organizations like Barnado's (Bloom 1968; Godek 1977; Reid 1979) and the National Children's Home (Payne 1979), to RCA Publications (Ollivant 1979) and the work of the National Children's Bureau (Page and Clark 1977). Otherwise we rely upon autobiographical material and novels.

This chapter attempts to show that despite the differences in age, circumstances, and destinations of children and young people leaving residential care, and despite the wide variety of needs this implies, there are common features to be recognized, acknowledged, and attended to by residential and community-based social workers responsible for their welfare.

For children 'in two minds' torn between feelings of stress, anxiety, and powerlessness on the one hand and on the other pleasure, hope, and optimism in the face of yet another ending and new beginning, the social work task will be to find means whereby a balance may be achieved, and the see-saw of ambivalence gradually weighted towards the positive: plus factors outweighing minus. The proposition pursued in this chapter is that if residential social work practice is to succeed, and children leaving residential care are to experience maximum life satisfaction and make the best possible use of the opportunities available to them wherever these may be, then it will be important that (1) they feel secure in a firm knowledge and understanding of their past and its influence upon their life, (2) they themselves participate in planning for their future, and (3) they be involved right now in preparations for departure, survival, and mastery on the assumption that leaving residential care will have been anticipated as part of the admission process and therefore that preparations for moving on will have begun already.

When they are to be received into care children want to know how long they can expect to stay and when they can expect to go home. By creating openings and talking about this at the earliest possible opportunity social workers establish a principle of honest exchange and mutual respect between children and the adult(s) with key responsibility for their welfare (RCA/BASW 1976). This will be essential for planning together towards the eventual outcome of a child's period in residence, whether it be return to parent(s) or not. Childhood is time-limited chronologically speaking, and it is inevitable that children will emerge from residential care eventually regardless of the original purpose/objectives of admission or the extent to which these have been realized and regardless of the quality of planning and review, or whether there has been adequate preparation for departure and after-care. Children emerge by virtue of the fact that they reach a particular point in time when they are deemed to have ceased to be children needing those things children are said to need (Pringle 1975). Thus, leaving residential care is inevitable for mentally alert, able-bodied young people – though it may be delayed in certain exceptional circumstances (Sereny 1974; Arden 1977). What is required of responsible creative social work practice is action on the basis of the recognition that time is precious in childhood, and that continuity of both experiences and relationships is crucial to healthy child development. Rowe and Lambert's study suggested that for children who had been in care for more than six months there was only a one in four chance of leaving before the age of sixteen; of the 2000 children studied one in four had moved three or more times, and the older the children the more moves they were likely to have made (1973). Fanshel and Shinn, in a longitudinal study over five years, found that the longer a child remained in care the more exposed he was to the possibility of being moved (1978). Thus, the right of a child to a permanent placement has become a matter of urgent concern (Adcock 1981).

The importance of counteracting drift, of exploring every possibility for a child, and securing the most propitious and least damaging living arrangement, given a comprehensive picture of his/her needs and circumstances, is well documented (Jehu 1963; Rowe and Lambert 1973; Shaw and Lebens 1978) and so too is how best to proceed (DHSS 1976a; ABAFA 1977, 1979). This chapter will concentrate instead upon what kinds of help can be offered to children and young people to ease their passage and prepare them to take their place in a new environment, be this family home, adoptive or foster home, digs, or another residential setting (Payne 1979) − and recognizing that there is another less conventional way of leaving residential care that warrants attention, namely absconding.

The focus for social work concern will be upon the child's perception of leaving, that mixture of hope and dread he experiences in anticipation; the focus for action will be upon those areas of a child's subjective and objective functioning which will need to be strengthened to ensure survival and mastery in a new environment. The direction and pace of intervention will be determined by the shifting degrees of confidence and competence that become apparent as work together proceeds towards departure and beyond. The objective will be to promote positive anticipation and a sense of secure investment in the future via joint planning and preparation that is anchored firmly to whatever realities the child will face when he leaves.

An attempt is made to identify common features; first, feelings and expectations which seem to be widely experienced and shared, and second issues which appear to be relevant to children of all ages, circumstances, and destinations who are leaving residential care; then, with proposition and common features in mind, some possibilities for social work in action are explored.

By finding ways of helping children to recognize and consolidate the good things in their past and present life and to accept and learn to live with the not so good; by ensuring that they anticipate the future as accurately as possible, that they are involved in the decision process and equipped to deal effectively both with the realities they will face and any associated fantasies; by using any and every opportunity here and now, in and around the residential setting, to engage them in preparation for leaving, together with peers and staff, it may be possible to minimize stresses and maximize the child's potential for turning the opportunities and pitfalls ahead to advantage.

What do we know about the feelings and expectations of children and young people leaving residential care? From a practice wisdom rich in empathy Stroud wrote in one of his novels:

'Royston had now been at Hawthorn Hill for two and a half years and he was almost fifteen. He often surprised himself with these facts; the years had gone by unnoticed. . . . After an initial period of panic at the thought of growing up, he experienced a fierce exhaltation, that he was finished with childhood, that soon he would be leaving school and leaving the Home. The idea filled him with something between pleasure and terror.'

(1963 : 108)

More recently young people themselves have provided direct evidence of this anxiety and ambivalence:

'At roughly the age of 16 it's brought home to you that there are only 2 more years to go before you are out. This gives rise to mixed feelings. On the one hand it's hip hip hooray – on the other there is fear of the unknown.'

(Page and Clark 1977:55)

Autobiographical accounts of leaving reveal mixed feelings too:

'Before I actually left the Home I started to spend one evening a week with my mother, I suppose to get to know her. . . . Those days spent with her made it startlingly clear what it was going to be like when I actually left, and it was with a great sense of sadness that I went to live with my mother, leaving behind friends and security to go again to a strange new home.'

(Timms 1973:51)

'The last day came; and I stood in my brand new clothes . . . I had not cried until the moment of parting . . . up till now, deep within me, I'd believed that something, someone would save me. . . . My tears were unremarked, for everyone cried when leaving the village, even if they had been miserable there . . . I just dumbly . . . went through the main gates to the tram leaving behind me that small, closed world that had for 3 years held all my dreams and shown me visions of life as it might be.'

(Hitchman 1966:180)

and:

'The time approached when I would be leaving. . . . It came much sooner than I'd anticipated . . . the Major had suggested that I should go to Reading where he could fix me up with a job and lodgings. I decided that this was what I would like to do. It really wasn't a very difficult decision to make because I had no friends in my home town . . . and there were two boys already living and working there . . . this could possibly be the break from my old ties that I'd been waiting for. . . . All in all it added up to a chance to make something out of the wreckage of my young life.'

(O'Neill 1981:45)

Leaving aside considerations such as differences in chrono-logical age and stage of social, emotional, and intellectual development, which will affect children's conception of time, space, and distance; their ability and willingness to think and plan ahead, and their powers of abstraction, not to mention sensitivity and capacity to tune in to their own and other people's feelings; and leaving aside the additional complicating factor of adolescence as a period of change and life crisis any-way, what features can be extracted as likely to be common to children and young people of any age, circumstances, and destination leaving residential care?

I would venture to suggest that the necessity of leaving resi-dential care and letting go – at any particular time – generates anxiety which in turn will affect a child's motivation for, and resistance to, change and transfer to a new environment. The nature of the anxiety experienced will depend to a large extent upon a particular child's personality, life history, and coping patterns, as well as upon factors mentioned as asides above, but it will depend also upon a core ingredient inherent to the event, namely ambivalence. Ambivalence in turn will be affected by the child's own particular perception of the gains to be made and the losses to be endured as a result of leaving. The social work task will be to use the group living situation, circum-stances, and resources to help children control their fears and fantasies and adjust their perception of things in order to face what will be the reality of leaving for each of them; to make it possible for them to participate in planning their own future, developing a sense of mastery over the direction of their lives so that planning and preparation for departure and afterwards brings with it a sense of investment in the outcome and of positive anticipation (Stoeffler 1972). Reminiscence will be the key tool for helping children to recall, reconstruct, conserve, and consolidate past and present, in communication with prac-titioners and peers, and establish firm foundations from which to move forward in life.

Fluctuating degrees of insecurity and denial must also be con-sidered. Again, the aim will be to reduce the need for denial and promote a greater sense of reality-based security. Where there has been no recovery from anxiety engendered by early separation, and where subsequent separations – with their accompanying reactions of loss and grief, protest and despair – have compounded the damage already done to a child's sense of valuing self and other people, then balance between motivation and resistance may become more difficult tó achieve. Ambivalence may become less apparent and the outcome may be an isolated, detached, self-absorbed loner who, given superficial social skills, veers towards extremes of independence rather than the dependence of those lacking adequate social skills or the healthy interdependence of 'people who need people' (*Figure 3(1)*).

From the mixed feelings and expectations common to children and young people leaving residential care – though experienced differentially – attention turns now to three groups of questions arising from the three elements of the original proposition. As represented below the proposition and allied questions offer a frame of reference from which to explore in more detail social work with children moving through a period of residence towards departure.

Successful outcomes for children and young people – their enthusiasm for, and ability to function in new settings and situations – will depend a great deal on the quality of social work input by adults with key responsibility for planning their future with them, reviewing progress, preparing for departure and for reception by the host environment, and maintaining subsequent supervision and support.

Whatever is anticipated, whether it is returning to parent(s), embarking upon life in a new family or residential unit, or going it alone, the objective will be to reduce negative anticipation and promote positive thought and action on the basis of a balanced perception of reality so that a youngster is in the best possible state of subjective and objective readiness to benefit from change.

Respecting children (Crompton 1980) demands amongst other things that practitioners attend to the questions, often unspoken, that bedevil the waking and sleeping hours of youngsters in residence. If children leaving residential care are to face both the opportunities and the pitfalls with confidence

Figure 3(1)

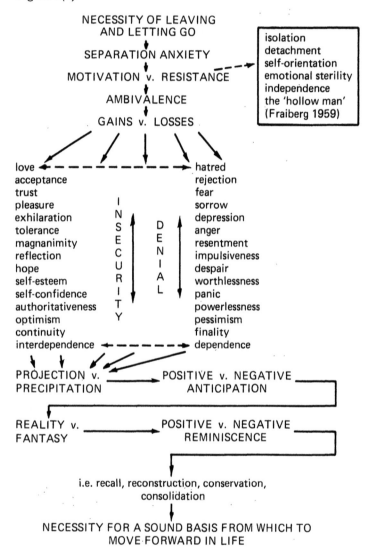

```
            NECESSITY OF LEAVING
              AND LETTING GO              ┌─────────────────────┐
                   │                      │ isolation           │
            SEPARATION ANXIETY            │ detachment          │
                   │                      │ self-orientation    │
          MOTIVATION v. RESISTANCE  ─ ─ ─►│ emotional sterility │
                   │                      │ independence        │
              AMBIVALENCE                 │ the 'hollow man'    │
                   │                      │ (Fraiberg 1959)     │
              GAINS v. LOSSES             └─────────────────────┘
```

love ◄ ─ ─ ─ ─ ─ ─ ─ ─ ─ ► hatred
acceptance   rejection
trust   fear
pleasure   I   sorrow
exhilaration   N   D   depression
tolerance   S   E   anger
magnanimity   E   N   resentment
reflection   C   I   impulsiveness
hope   U   A   despair
self-esteem   R   L   worthlessness
self-confidence   I   panic
authoritativeness T   powerlessness
optimism   Y   pessimism
continuity   finality
interdependence ◄ ─ ─ ─ ─ ► dependence

PROJECTION v. ─────────► POSITIVE v. NEGATIVE
PRECIPITATION   ANTICIPATION

REALITY v. ─────────► POSITIVE v. NEGATIVE
FANTASY   REMINISCENCE

        i.e. recall, reconstruction, conservation,
                    consolidation

     NECESSITY FOR A SOUND BASIS FROM WHICH TO
                MOVE FORWARD IN LIFE
i.e. secure identity, positive self-image, confidence, and competence

and competence, then, assuming that leaving is anticipated as part of the admission process and the issue kept alive, three preliminaries will be important.

(1) A SECURE KNOWLEDGE AND UNDERSTANDING OF THE PAST

'A social worker is there to help you understand and to tell you the truth. If we're in care, and it's our lives, we have a right to know what's going on in our lives and why our parents can't have us home. . . . For all you know they might be dead. Like A. said, all the time he was growing up in care he thought his parents were dead, but when he got out he found that they were both alive.'

(Page and Clark 1977:33)

(2) PARTICIPATION IN PLANNING FOR THEIR OWN FUTURE

'I think the Council's got "rights and powers" over me but I'm not sure what that means.'

(Page and Clark 1977:31)

'many adults do not think of children as having the right to (or the ability for) active involvement in their own destinies and development.'

(Wardle 1975)

(3) CONTINUOUS INVOLVEMENT IN PREPARATION FOR LEAVING

'I want to know where I'm going to be living and what's going to happen to me. I've been in so many different places.'

(Page and Clark 1977:29)

'When I was fostered, I hadn't even met the foster parents. I wasn't even told I was going there until they said "Put your coat on we're going." '

(p. 46)

'I'm not prepared . . . I don't know how I will manage, I can't even boil an egg.'

(p. 53)

'I won't have any friends when I leave care.'

(p. 54)

Children and young people seem to be saying that they are precipitated out of residential care, ill-prepared psychologically and practically, insufficiently kitted out for survival let alone mastery in a new environment. In other words the following questions go unanswered.

(1) Secure knowledge and understanding of the past

Who am I?
What am I (role(s))?
Where am I; how did I get here; and where was I before?
Where is everyone?
Why am I here; how long will I stay?
What's supposed to happen whilst I'm here and what's expected of me?

Focus and Direction of Social Work Task

IDENTITY CRISIS	↗	JUSTIFIABLE SELF-ABSORPTION	↗	SELF IN CONTEXT	↗	OTHER CONSCIOUSNESS (or altruism)

(2) Participation in planning the future

Where am I going (general)?
Why?
Is it what I want?
Are there any alternatives?
What are they and what would they mean for/demand of me, and the people who are important to me?
Who has the power to influence matters?
Do I have any say?
If so, how do I go about it and who will support me?

Focus and Direction of Social Work Task

LACK OF INFLUENCE/ CONTROL OVER EVENTS	POWERLESSNESS and DISAFFECTION	INFLUENCE/ CONTROL OVER LIFE CHOICES	INVESTMENT IN OUTCOME(S)
↗	↗	↗	

(3) Involvement in preparation for departure and after

Where am I going (specific)?
How will I get there?
Who will I meet and what will they expect of me?

What will I need $\begin{cases} \text{to be} \\ \text{to know} \\ \text{to have} \\ \text{to do} \end{cases}$ in order to cope?

Will I be equipped, psychologically, materially?

? Will I be able to manage $\begin{cases} \text{myself} \\ \text{my money} \\ \text{my school work (job)} \\ \text{relationships with my own and the} \\ \quad \text{opposite sex} \\ \text{relationships with strangers and} \\ \quad \text{with my own family} \end{cases}$

Who can I turn to for help and support?
Can I keep in touch?
What happens if I fail?
Is there any way back?
? Will I be able to get/keep control over my own life

choices, i.e. $\begin{cases} \text{job} \\ \text{partner} \\ \text{lifestyle} \end{cases}$

? What will I be $\begin{cases} \text{attractive, rich, famous, autonomous,} \\ \quad \text{and loved} \\ \qquad\qquad\qquad \text{or} \\ \text{unemployed, stigmatized, disregarded,} \\ \text{discriminated against, and friendless} \end{cases}$

Focus and Direction of Social Work Task

INSUFFICIENT practical, social, economic, and political KNOWLEDGE: social and practical SKILLS	↗	practical, social, economic, and political HELPLESSNESS and VULNERABILITY	↗	COMPETENCE and CONFIDENCE born of appropriate and functional KNOWLEDGE and SKILLS	↗	S U R V I V A L	M A S T E R Y

IDENTITY: THE TASKS

Successful outcomes for children may depend upon the ability of key workers to involve parents and parenting persons as full and equal partners in the process of planning, review (Gutridge 1980), and preparation for departure. All too often, however, parents have been lost to children and I propose to proceed with this in mind.

> 'government reports, legislation and research studies . . . support the . . . belief that the family is the most important influence on a child's life and should be preserved for him even at great cost in resources and effort. But somehow, somewhere the decision to preserve the family of these children, or to provide substitute parents, had not been taken.'
>
> (Lasson 1981:14)
>
> '(nevertheless) natural parents remain of primary importance whether there is contact or not.'
>
> (p. 49)
>
> '(and) . . . lack of resolution of strong feelings towards natural parents was a disturbing feature of (my) study.'
>
> (p. 50)

Learning the truth about yourself, your family background, and your journey through life to date can be painful but not to know can be more so (ABAFA 1976; DHSS 1976a; Day 1980; Triseliotis 1980). To a child whose sense of self has become fragmented by separation and loss the need for information and for help with digesting that information and incorporating it as part of the self-image is great; but what is it that children need to know, how is the knowledge mislaid, and what can be done? Children's knowledge about themselves depends a great deal upon other people's knowledge of them and how possible it is to retrieve that knowledge once stored, in mind or on paper; on the readiness of adults to recognize and appreciate the importance of the knowledge they possess, to share and discuss it; and on how available they are to a child as time passes.

Two kinds of information are important for a child: that which concerns significant people, places, and events in his life (such as when, why, and how he came into care, what happened to parents, siblings, and other relatives, where the child has been since, with whom, for how long, and in what sequence), and information about the child's own self that is essentially personal and marks his uniqueness.

Information is lost because children move about, and so do the adults who care for them. Parts of a child's self may be lost in places long forgotten and with people long gone. When significant people are lost to children so too are a mass of memories and minutiae about them which are profoundly precious – anecdotes and idiosyncracies, fads and folklore – which the continuity of family life would normally protect and keep in trust; bits of a child's identity which are unique and woven into a pattern which is reflected back to him over the years indicating who he is, where he belongs, and what he is like. Lasson suggests that a sense of continuity and history is lost because the child does not share his daily life with anyone who can recall what he was like a few years ago, reminisce with him, or polish his image of his early years; and because there is no one to remember with him such occasions as losing his first tooth, taking his first steps, and his first day at school (1981:9–10). To lose what is particular to you at such times – as perceived by adults who care for you – impoverishes children in ways that perhaps are little appreciated. Like dropping toys over the side of the pram and having them reliably returned, the security that comes from salvaged memories is incalculable.

The extent to which the lost parts of a child's self can be

retained and recovered may be the extent to which his sense of wholeness as a person can be assured. Consequently when children, or staff, expect to move perhaps efforts should be made to preserve in trust these privileged, exclusive recollections about a child so often irretrievably locked away in the minds and hearts of residential (and field) staff who have shared children's lives for a time. These could be stored in writing, in picture book form, or on tape to aid crucial reminiscence; pieces of the jigsaw puzzle to be reconstructed gradually and appreciated at leisure; a means of reordering the pack of cards tossed in the air so long ago and fallen who knows where. Compiling this store of recollections together could be a constructive means of helping children deal with feelings about losing valued adults and of strengthening their capacity to cope with similar events in future.

The need to piece together the past and make sense of it is reflected in Tom O'Neill's account of his brother Terry's efforts in adulthood to retrace his steps and reconstruct past events so as to find some peace of mind and be able to get on with living in the here and now (O'Neill 1981).

Conserving parts of a child's self means more than people, places, and events. Objects and belongings have significance too. A piece of clothing, a toy, a postcard, or photo may be a vital link with the past. Yet a child can become bereft of such items in residential care either because there is nowhere private to keep belongings, and they are lost or misappropriated, or because they seem unimportant and no one thinks ahead for the child and gathers them up for safe keeping (Jones 1970).

Vigilance about keeping objects that are, or may be, significant to a child and engaging children's interest, understanding, and co-operation in this may pay dividends later. For example, keeping such objects as birthday and postcards from a mum who may disappear; cloth comforters used when sucking one's thumb; toys and story books brought from home and old teddies who came into care at the same time; items of clothing bought by a relative and long outgrown and discarded; pictures painted at school and modelling creations fleetingly admired but which a parent might have lovingly retained; trophies and certificates won; old school reports and exercise books; photographs of people, places, and events, and of oneself at different ages; letters and postcards from individuals who may play a key part in some later reconstruction. It will be important not to defeat the object of the exercise by whipping away belongings prematurely or, in excess of zeal, imposing practices on children which instead of helping become additional sources of anxiety. In theory, however, nothing that may have associations and strike a vital chord later is too petty or bizarre to be included. Decisions about what is to be held in safe keeping, when, where, and for how long, and matters of access, would be negotiable as part of the working relationship between child and key worker (RCA/BASW 1976).

When it comes to exploring together ways of reconstructing the past, correcting misconceptions, and filling in gaps – perhaps making scrapbooks, or life maps, or writing (or taping) a dramatized autobiography – then objects held in trust that otherwise might have been lost can be used to assist recall and reappraisal (Pharis 1967; ABAFA, 1977, 1979). Agency records too may be a valuable source of material for helping in this respect. Parents' letters to the agency and correspondence that has been gathering dust on file for years may contain descriptions of family circumstances prior to admission, reasons for giving up the child, expressions of distress, regret, and hope for the child's future, plus clear evidence of positive and loving thoughts about their child. Extracted from the file (leaving a photocopy), used in discussion together, and given to a youngster to keep, letters in a parent's handwriting can have tremendous emotional significance and healing properties for those long out of touch with their family of origin. Photos too may be discovered in old files, and graphic cameos of recording by previous social workers recapturing times past and resurrecting for a child mental images of people and places that have long become blurred.

However theoretically desirable it may be for children and young people to see what is written about them, open access to files would be unrealistic whilst the purposes for which records are kept, and the principles and methods of compilation and storage, remain unchanged. Even selective access under the current system(s) presents problems (Timms 1972). What is advocated is selective use of existing material to the advantage of children and young people in residential care in the belief that this is a resource largely untapped; also that a record be kept of what children have been told, how, by whom, and under what circumstances, and of the child's reactions. The same factual information may be repeated time and again, and a child may accumulate several marginally conflicting interpretations unless staff are scrupulous about recording exchanges with children for reference by colleagues.

With the focus and direction of social work tasks in mind, residential social workers will be seeking opportunities for preserving and reconstructing the past with children alongside the essential routines of daily life in the residential setting. Everyday life continues unabated and whilst engaged in all manner of activities key workers will remain alive to children's questions, thoughts, and feelings, ready to tune in and develop tentative beginnings or create openings for discussion, checking whether this or that is significant to a child or not, ready to help a child to work backwards in order to move forwards (Britton 1955). Key workers bridge gaps for children between people, places, and events, between fact (the external world) and fantasy (the child's feelings about it). Expressions of thought and feeling open the door to a child's inner world and key workers 'will try to recognise and tune into the little pieces of the iceberg visible on the surface to help the child handle realities however painful and digest them emotionally'. We know that images become blurred for children by associated feelings of rejection and guilt, anger, fear, and misery. The social work task will be to help children hold onto reality and keep it relatively unclouded by fantasy by listening for casual remarks, symbolic stories, and apparently innocent questions whose true meanings are embedded in a particular child's life context, and by being deft enough in using such opportunities as they arise to shape children's emotional development (Winnicott 1964).

Group encounters in residential settings are rich in opportunities. Groups may be informal or consciously formalized, open or closed; a group baking in the kitchen or servicing the minibus out front may be doing just that but also be engaged upon deep and wide-ranging life topics, learning as much about self, and self in relation to others, as about the jobs in hand; impromptu bathroom and sitting-room groups may be spurred into profound examinations of 'life, the universe and everything', whilst well-established bedroom groups may be enormously supportive in enabling one another to explore painful memories and experiences productively. A problem shared may not necessarily be a problem halved but the success of the 'Who Cares?' groups is just one example of the potential value for children in residence of focused group discussion under sensitive participatory guidance (Page and Clark 1977), and of the potential for liberating education.

Staff and children will be doing more than travelling parallel lines alongside one another day to day. Locked into shared living, residential social workers engage with children in working at life so that, rather than being at the mercy of their inner and outer worlds, they gain a measure of understanding and control, and begin to be able to think more clearly about their lives.

'first we try to reach the child, establish communication and construct a working relationship which is personal yet structured. Having reached the child we try to look at his world with him and to help him to sort out his feelings about it: to face the painful things and to discover the good things. Then we try to consolidate the positive things in the child himself and in his world, and help him to make the most of his life.

(Winnicott 1964:57)

To be in residential work and to operate one-dimensionally, focusing only on the external world of chores and routine would be to miss the wonderland 'through the looking glass' where the real work with children moving through residence lies.

PARTICIPATION: THE TASKS

Lee and Pithers (1980), writing about radical residential child care, point out that residential work has not been without its radicals trying to counteract the primitive, controlling, and containing functions of residential living. Wills, for example, worked on the principle that if you treat young people with love and respect, share responsibility with them, and regard them as intelligent, then they will become more 'complete'; that an attitude of responsibility towards, and accountability to, the 'living community', once established and internalized, would be transferred to society as a whole. Each individual in Wills's care was cherished in his individuality and encouraged in his responsibility to others. Taking us beyond liberal therapeutic tradition to contemporary practice the authors draw attention to a list of aims drawn up by a Socialist Child Care Collective for a children's community day centre in London and which might be applied to residential child care (1975).

For residential social workers concerned to ensure that children participate in planning their future, prepare realistically for departure, and get the best possible deal out of life, these aims are of particular interest and although analysis of the aims and of the theoretical perspective from which they originate is beyond my brief, a statement of them here may add a helpful dimension to what follows. The aims are:

(1) To challenge competition and individualism.
(2) To develop group awareness and interdependence.
(3) To build up the self-confidence and interdependence of each child so that they can take their full part in the group.
(4) To break down hierarchies.
(5) To challenge the domination of the weak by the strong.
(6) To break down stereotyped sex roles.
(7) To develop warm emotional relationships not exclusive to the nuclear family.
(8) To develop an understanding of political questions; and Lee and Pithers make an addition of their own, namely
(9) To combat racism.

It is my view that children have a right to be heard, that they should know that they have this right, and be encouraged to use it to good effect.

'I've never been to my review. I've asked but they won't let me.'

(Page and Clark 1977:42)

'I think all kids should have the chance to say what they want to happen to them and where they are going to go when they leave.'

(p. 42)

Whilst choice is important with regard to attending formal reviews, enabling children to participate in other ways in planning and deciding about their own future will be vital. Ensuring knowledge and understanding of what has happened already in their lives cannot be divorced from open speculation about what is to come. Children will need to know about the alternatives, and they will need help to appreciate the implications of these and what each alternative might mean to them or require of them. Most of the work can be done together long before reviews or case conferences convene to formalize matters and make decisions. Key worker and child can explore together what is possible, and preferred, and how desired outcomes might be achieved. For those who do not wish to attend, their key worker can continue to act as mediator and advocate, but where children and young people do attend and participate, practitioners will want to ensure that they know where the power lies and who has the final say, and that they know the ropes. In other words, apart from asking children their views and making sure they have the necessary information and understanding on which to base an opinion, apart from listening to their replies, respecting their position and acting as advocate, it will be of vital importance to teach children how to handle themselves in reviews so that they know what, and who, to expect, how to respond to questions, present their case, and do themselves justice. Rehearsal in the form of group role play of review and case conference situations may not only help to advance their cause and improve their social skills, it may also reduce tension and anxiety and save them pain (Page and Clark 1977).

The aftermath and anticlimax of formal reviews and case

discussions are seldom appreciated and the importance of opportunities for children to reflect upon what has happened cannot be overestimated. It might help if review panels produced some form of simple statement committed to paper on the spot with a copy for everyone concerned to take away with them, including the child. This would provide something visible, a reference point and working tool for child and worker(s) alike. In some instances written submission by the child might be of value, providing a record of his contributions and pattern of his thinking over time to which he and the worker could refer. Too much responsibility however could be overwhelming and defeat its own purpose, inducing anxiety and insecurity rather than their more positive counterparts. Participation is not meant to imply full responsibility for decision-making (see Page and Clark 1977:30).

If things do not go the way a youngster has hoped, then the aftermath of review, and staying with him in reflection and adjustment, will be especially important.

Without denying the inequality of a child's situation in relation to the authority of staff and agency hierarchy, what is advocated is dialogue and negotiation between children and those with responsibility for their welfare, and some form of liberating education, so that whilst they are still in relatively protected circumstances they can learn to reckon with social and practical realities relating to their age or sex or colour, or their prospects in the labour market, and to negotiate acceptably and effectively on their own behalf.

When there is no opportunity to participate or to engage in dialogue and negotiation, then there may be little investment in any particular outcome and a child may take unilateral action and run away. This may be one of the few ways for a child in residential care to exercise self-determination, and convey to surrounding adults what for some reason could not be communicated in any other way.

Absconding has been ill understood and little studied, and too often it seems as if field and residential social workers respond on the basis of self-interest and self-protection instead of questioning the meaning of the child's behaviour in relation to themselves and their efforts on the child's behalf. To be fair, runaway children usually provoke mixed feelings – guilt, anger, and fear for the child's safety – all of which may confuse the issue and prevent attention being focused upon the child's predicament and distress, and why he ran off.

> 'C. did a bunk at least once a fortnight, pathetically but determinedly trying to get home to his mum. He was about 7 or 8 and he was nearly always caught the day after bunking and returned issuing tears and pledges never to do it again to the stern Gaffer.'

> (Thomas 1967:137)

Punishment and constraint may mollify staff and subdue children but achieve little else and certainly not a better understanding between children and adults.

Farrington *et al.* (1968) identify half a dozen patterns amongst groups of runaway children:

(1) Where sudden crisis led to severe panic reaction and fright.
(2) Where children, whose basic reaction to stress was withdrawal and who found it difficult to adjust to residential care, drifted off in aimless retreat.
(3) Where behaviour seemed to be directly related to a child's past and present relationships with family, and the key may be some link between past home experiences and present 'in residence' experiences, for example when a child finds himself 'piggy in the middle' between adults in conflict.
(4) Where an experience of loss in the present (key worker leaving) triggers the child's incapacity to handle separation and loss.
(5) Where the child fears something is wrong at home, that he is needed and must be there to ward off disaster; and
(6) Where children are locked into a never-ending search for lost parents.

Perhaps one could add at least one other category ie:

(7) Where children are dissatisfied, despondent, and powerless yet spirited enough to draw attention to their plight directly

either on impulse or as the consequence of a planned series of unilateral actions. 'When I ran away I felt, well, somebody's got to do something if I run away, so I did' (Kahan 1979:140).

Farrington *et al.* (1968) advocate a therapeutic rather than a punitive response, and using the runaway behaviour to help a child clarify his situation, his relationships, and his life options. This envisages welcoming the maverick home with loving relief and an evident concern to try to understand, and put things to rights.

Whatever the pattern, running away appears to be a means of communicating distress. As such it presents yet another opportunity to invite a child to develop a sense of investment in his own future by participating in a realistic appraisal of his situation and in forward planning.

PREPARATION FOR DEPARTURE AND AFTERWARDS:
THE TASKS

Objective criteria for judging the readiness of children or young people to leave a particular residential establishment and move on are difficult to identify, and decisions are prey to subjectivity of staff and case conferences, but an important consideration in negotiating a departure and its timing will be what the child wants, given the alternatives available, and how he perceives the issues to be faced prior to leaving and immediately afterwards.

Childhood is a dynamic, inexorable process of change and development, physical, emotional, intellectual, and perceptual in terms of a sense of identity, and subjective and objective worth. Ideally change occurs within the security of a familiar constant world peopled by consistent trusted adults who also remain constant. Despite criticism of the nuclear family as ideal (Cooper 1972) the fact remains that it is this ideal to which children in care aspire, as their fantasies would seem to confirm (Hart 1977). For children in residence the usual settings for natural growth and development have been disrupted, perhaps lost to them altogether, and as departure approaches it is accompanied by a foreboding magnified beyond the average.

Lasson (1981) found that thirty years after the Curtis Report, which criticized the separateness of institutions from their surrounding neighbourhood, and many other reports stressing the importance of integration into the community, staff and children still referred to 'the Outside' (p. 41) and very few children had even limited involvement with families or organizations in the area of the home. She points out that meeting other children and their parents would seem to be an area of experience of particular value in preparing for adult roles, or indeed for the role of adoptive or foster child, and she asserts that a necessary part of the residential task must be to enable children and young people to build a wider network of significant people in their lives, and to develop the skills necessary for making new relationships and learning new roles. Unless the surrounding community is seen and used as a prime resource social work tasks cannot be fulfilled and the proposition falls.

'(Children) are not adequately prepared for adult life and most express strong fears as their time to meet adulthood draws near. Only a handful have their mother or father nearby to help . . . and the SSD will have no legal obligation when they've passed their 18th birthday . . . Staff are more optimistic however and seem unaware of some of the children's deep seated fears.'

(Lasson 1981:47)

It may be that an air of finality about leaving on the threshold of adulthood accentuates other elements of negative anticipation, putting the outcome at greater risk than might otherwise be so given a flexible approach.

'At the end, there was the gate to the Outside, and it opened for each of us, opened only once. Its notice, hung on its top bar, said "Shut the Gate Behind You" which was an instruction as final as any.'

(Thomas 1967:171)

Being able to stay on beyond eighteen is one means of combating finality, staggered transition is another, and also being able to return in the event of initial failure.

'20/25 children of all ages presently live at Mill Grove and there is no prescribed leaving age. Those at work may have their own bed sitters on the premises . . . and whilst eventually most leave the building a high proportion remain in contact for the rest of their lives.'

(White 1980:28)

'One of our family is nearly 20. He works in a bank. On account of a tragic event in his family his early years were separated from his present experience of himself yet by becoming more and more an older brother/uncle to some younger children he has started to relive his early years. This is the sort of healing process that a varied community makes possible.'

(p. 31)

Children returning home, or moving out into substitute families, will want to do so gradually, to know that they can keep in touch and that their bed will still be there for them if they need it. Teenagers too need to know that there is a bolt-hole and that they are not cut off entirely but can return to visit, stay over, or retreat when things get too much for them.

Following children out of residential care will be essential, for to truncate the process of admission to residence, throughput, and after-care is to place the outcome for a child or young person gravely at risk. Preparation for departure, departure itself, and provision for continuing care, attention, and support in the new environment cannot be separated one from another. Just as the process cannot be truncated without harm being caused, close working relationships between key workers and children cannot be summarily severed without despoiling what they have shared and achieved together, without impoverishing a child's future and placing in peril his chances of successful adjustment and steady progress towards a broader inter-dependence. A continuing relationship and involvement with his key worker(s) beyond the boundaries of residential living and into the wider community aims to provide crucial bridges between past, present, and future and to ensure overall continuity of experience whether children are returning home, joining new families, or facing the world as beginning adults. Children moving into foster homes, or those for whom an agency retains some other statutory responsibility, will be assured of continuing social work support. Social work practice in adoption is sensitive to the continuing needs of adoptees and adopters, especially where older and handicapped children and sibling groups reveal special needs. Thus it is the beginning adults who are at greatest risk of being left to sink or swim on leaving residential care.

Accounts of the work of Barnado's in the last decade or so reveal a rich variety of efforts made to counteract the risk of loneliness, depression, and failure long-witnessed amongst youngsters out on their own, and to increase chances of success. These include halfway houses, hostels, and bed-sit accommodation, staffed and unstaffed; special foster homes; self-contained annexes to children's homes; single rooms and other privileged facilities for older children; study bedrooms for sixth form and higher education students, and apprentices; also youth groups and clubs; reunions and newsletters; continuing social work support out in the community; and the maintenance of close, supportive, often pseudo-parental links with residential and field staff long after departure (Bloom 1968; Gutridge 1970; Godek 1977; Reid 1979).

What is important is not so much the provision of accommodation and facilities for young people as the opportunities these create for staff to help youngsters prepare for adult life, to ensure continuing support for them and a gradual weaning from dependence upon the agency and its social workers paced to each youngster's needs. Reid points to the importance of recognizing possible difficulties at an early stage and planning carefully with those youngsters who will have to make their own homes on leaving residential care, and she goes on to describe her own group-work efforts and training programme (Reid 1979). What emerges from these accounts and from Godek's study (1977) is that children need to be more involved in the daily running of residential establishments in order to help them to be able to define basic household and other essential tasks. With help they can then identify the knowledge and skill they will require in order to fulfil these tasks and set about acquiring them before they leave, so gaining competence and confidence in advance. The importance of instilling hope of achievement and mastery cannot be overstated (Smaldino 1975). Because of the nature of adolescence (Coleman 1980), and the significance of peer culture (Vorrath and Brendtro 1974), learning together in groups has particular value (Gutridge 1970; Reid 1979), perhaps by practical demonstrations and experiment (cooking, repairs) or role play exercises (visiting the Job Centre) in a climate of fun and achievement.

Since adolescence is a time of accelerated change (La Barre 1969), a time for the tasks of extricating oneself from dependent childhood and establishing a separate and more settled identity (Erikson 1965; Rayner 1971), admired adults may well be idealized as models for how or what a young person would like to become (Russian 1975). Harnessed and used with care by key workers this susceptibility to idealization and modelling may help staff to engage youngsters in preparatory tasks before leaving and then to encourage continuation of their efforts and development of their skills and confidence as part of an after-care programme. Social work with young people leaving residential care is about promoting feelings of self-worth and adequacy, providing a second chance to reflect upon and sort out feelings about the past, helping them to tackle tasks and fulfil roles that are important to them so that rather than barely surviving they can learn to master their new environment and carve a life-style for themselves that will enable them to make life choices that will benefit both themselves and others.

Objectives and related tasks at the stages of preparation for departure and afterwards will include (1) promoting the acquisition of knowledge, and practical and interpersonal skills; (2) securing certain practical provision; (3) safeguarding personal possessions and ensuring that these accompany the child or young person when he leaves; (4) considering the appropriateness or otherwise of ceremonies to mark his passage; (5) supporting him in transition from A to B; and (6) consolidating and developing his knowledge and skills, competence and confidence. as he establishes himself in his new environment.

Figure 3(2) enlarges upon these suggestions and, without intending to represent definitive lists, attempts to demonstrate the significance of after-care. Fulfilling social work tasks cannot be confined to the period in residence but must assume continuation of working relationships between key workers and children/young people well beyond departure. The length of time required for the after-care of young people is impossible to specify and must be paced to meet the needs of the individual. What is certain, however, is that the absence of planned follow-up and after-care, so integral to the social work process in hand, will mean diminishing returns from previous social work input.

Figure 3(2) Preparation for departure and afterwards

SOCIAL WORK TASKS

(A) to promote acquisition of KNOWLEDGE about e.g.

    (1) the cost of living

    (2) the job and accommodation markets

    (3) social, economic, and political realities

    (4) achieving a balanced diet

    (5) budgeting and management of money

        rent and overheads, food
        household articles
        clothing and toiletries
        personal items – make-up, cigarettes, records/tapes, books/maps, sports and other equipment

    (6) saving and investment

    (7) rights and responsibilities of an employee (NI contributions, sickness benefits, etc.)

    (8) sexual encounter and its responsibilities

    (9) basic health care and first-aid (in case of illness or injury)

    (10) the elementary workings of household amenities (electrical, water, waste, and heating systems)

    (11) community services and resources

    (12) what to do in an emergency (accident, fire, theft, who to contact and how, etc.)

(B) to promote acquisition of PRACTICAL SKILLS e.g.

    (1) how to shop for, prepare, and cook food

    (2) how to maintain personal hygiene

Figure 3(2)—*cont.*

    (3) how to go about simple household repairs

        mending a fuse
        changing plugs and light bulbs
        replacing a washer

    (4) sewing and mending − buttons, hems, zips, etc.
    (5) how to find and use community services and resources
    (6) how, when and where to find their own, or another, social worker/caring agency

(C) to promote acquisition of SOCIAL AND INTERPERSONAL SKILLS e.g.

    (1) initiating relationships and making friends
    (2) sustaining relationships
    (3) terminating, surviving, and recovering from relationships
    (4) interaction in one-to-one, and group situations in a variety of circumstances; male, female, or mixed company, young or old(er)
    (5) interaction and negotiation with

        adoptive, or foster, parents − their children and
          relatives
        landlords and landladies
        employers and fellow employees
        DHSS and other officials
        police
        doctors
        teachers
        social workers
        friends and neighbours

(D) to secure PRACTICAL PROVISION e.g.

    (1) new clothes/wardrobe − negotiated to reflect child or young person's choices and preferences plus practical requirements
    (2) bedding
    (3) furniture and furnishings
    (4) household articles
    (5) alarm clock

(E) to safeguard PERSONAL POSSESSIONS and ensure that these accompany the child/young person when he leaves e.g.

    (1) post office savings book
    (2) passport
    (3) medical card
    (4) birth certificate

Figure 3(2)—*cont.*
    (5) national insurance card
    PLUS
        familiar clothing
        appliances − transistor radio, record player, hair dryer,
        rollers, tongs, electric shavers, etc.
        precious books and toys
        school reports
        trophies and certificates
        photos, memorabilia
        musical instruments
        sports equipment
        pets
(F) if/when appropriate/desired to arrange CEREMONIES to mark the
    passage of a child/young person e.g.
        (1) parties − with perhaps cards and/or gifts exchanged, discos
        (2) special outings − theatre, ballet, pop concerts, etc.
(G) to support him IN TRANSITION e.g.
        helping him to move in, rearrange himself and his posses-
        sions, establish preliminary contacts, begin work or training,
        etc.
(H) to consolidate and develop knowledge and skills, COMPETENCE and
    CONFIDENCE via
        continuing attention to (A), (B), (C), and (D).

Children in Lasson's study (1981) who reported angry, sad
feelings ranked their parents as most important to them despite
the fact that they became more isolated from their roots as they
grew older. Those who reported happy, relaxed feelings ranked
their house parent(s) first. In Lasson's view those children who
had been able to transfer warm feelings for parents to key
workers (without betrayal) were more positive in outlook whilst
those who could not remained detached and hostile. It follows
therefore that outcomes for children and young people will
depend upon input; and that less painful and more successful
transition from residential care will be related to the quality of
social work practice from the process of admission, through a
child's period in residence, to the point of departure and
beyond.

4   Handicapped Children
Elizabeth Tarran

In *Living with Handicap* Younghusband *et al.* (1970) defined
handicap as 'a disability which for a substantial period, or
permanently, retards, distorts or otherwise adversely affects
normal growth, development or adjustment to life'. This definition has become quite widely accepted since, as for example in
the Court Report (DHSS 1976b). Mitchell (in Drillien and
Drummond 1977:1) highlighted the significance of a child's
home background: 'social deprivation and an inadequate home
and parents tend to increase handicap whereas it is lessened by a
warm supportive family. Thus a child's strengths and weaknesses, the resources and deficiencies of his home background,
and the impact of his surrounding environment must all be considered in determining the degree of his handicap.' In this sense
disability can then only be considered a handicap in relation to
circumstances. The social worker's contribution can be to
minimize the negative and reinforce and enhance the positive
effects of the individual circumstances of the child, thus
minimizing the overall handicap.

The amount of handicap in a community is difficult to
measure as what constitutes a handicap in one may not do so in
another and the degree of a child's handicap varies according to
his environment. Kirman (1972:13) said 'mental handicap is
not really a thing in itself but involves the notion of how society
reacts to its less able citizens'. To estimate its prevalence begs
the question of which handicaps, and to what degree of severity,
should be included. Pless and Pinkerton (1975) considered that
children with chronic illness or disability comprise at least 5–10
per cent of the population under the age of sixteen. Should these
children with chronic illness be regarded as handicapped? It is

possible that they experience hospitalization or periods of residence in care in a similar way to others who are more clearly defined as handicapped. Bradshaw (1975) estimated that there were between 85–108 thousand children with very severe mental and/or physical disability in Britain (i.e. 0.8 per cent of the childhood population). From this estimate, Mitchell (1977) extrapolated that there were maybe three to four thousand seriously handicapped children in the country or about 3 per cent of the population. This extrapolation was based on the assumption that there are about three moderately severely affected children for every one very severely affected. In about two-thirds of the seriously handicapped children, mental retardation is the major or only disability.

Most recent research studies relate largely to a particular type or degree of handicap, thus giving rates for each type. For this chapter the definition of Younghusband *et al.* (1970) will be used, thus the estimates given in the Court Report (DHSS 1976b) may be more meaningful to the practising social worker. These estimates, derived from reliable published survey reports, were applied to the average health district having approximately 60,000 children between 0–16 years (3750 in each yearly age group). It was suggested that:

'about 1,125 children aged 0–4 years will be moderately or severely handicapped by either physical (somatic), motor, visual, hearing and communication, or learning disorders which require special health care; 140 of them might need to attend special school, full- or part-time, according to their age. About 4,125 children of compulsory school age will be similarly handicapped. Of these 700 might need to attend special schools . . . these are approximate numbers.'

(DHSS 1976b : 220)

Social handicap was excluded, as was psychiatric disorder, as neither are in themselves intrinsic functional handicaps, but adverse social factors also occur frequently in the many children who are slightly or moderately handicapped. A social work contribution is then likely to enhance the lives of handicapped children and their families, regardless of the type and severity of handicap.

In order to best understand what social work methods and processes are most appropriate for use when working with handicapped children and their families when the child is leaving residential care, we must first look at how policy regarding residential care provision has developed. This should permit a greater understanding of the very varied provision that can constitute, for a handicapped child, the experience of residential care and can give some indication of the types and numbers of children using these different facilities. It will also permit some exploration of the differential effects of certain types of institution. Focusing on past and present trends and concepts in care provision will go some way towards understanding the reasons behind the need for residential care. A close examination of the particular circumstances that precipitate individual children's admissions will then enable clearer thinking about the meaning of the period of residence and how this will affect both the child and his family on discharge. Consideration can then be given to the particular needs, problems, and experiences that are likely to be encountered by the child and his family at the point of leaving residential care and shortly afterwards. Bearing in mind these needs and problems, we can then select the methods of work and information we require as social workers to bring a positive contribution to children and families who are undergoing a new experience that may be potentially stressful or even traumatic.

THE DEVELOPMENT OF CARE AND TREATMENT FOR THE HANDICAPPED CHILD

Until the 1950s little consideration had been given to caring for handicapped children in any way other than a residential institution catering for all ages and degrees of handicap. However, as more attention was paid to the needs of normal children, gradually handicapped children began to be considered too. By the end of the decade the concept of 'community care' was being recommended in the Mental Health Act 1959, giving local health authorities powers to provide day and residential services for children and adults.

The Platt Report (Central Health Services Council 1959) gave an additional boost to the consideration of the needs, particularly emotional, of children in hospital. The Brooklands Experiment (Tizard 1964) highlighted the effects that different patterns of management, environment, and staffing can have on the behaviour and performance of severely mentally handicapped young children. In a small, homelike unit, children did measurably better than controls in a large, long-stay hospital.

Within the next few years the Children and Young Person's Act 1963 and the Local Authority Social Service Act 1970 were concerned with the needs of children with regard both to the organizational structure and powers of local authority social services. However, within the hospitals a series of investigations began into the system of caring for mentally handicapped people after allegations of ill-treatment and other irregularities at specific hospitals. The first report, about Ely Hospital, Cardiff (Cmnd. 3957), made it clear that the concept of community care had been insufficiently developed (DHSS 1969). In response, the Secretary of State for Social Services began energetically to promote community care policies. Also a study by Morris (1969) financed by the National Society for Mentally Handicapped Children contributed much evidence to the case for reorganization of services.

Oswin (1971) in a study financed by the Spastics Society brought to public attention the plight of chronically handicapped children living permanently in institutions. Also in 1971, a detailed statement of government policy was published, having been delayed by a general election leading to a Tory government taking power, with different policies. This White Paper entitled 'Better Services for the Mentally Handicapped' (DHSS/Welsh Office 1971) proposed a shift to a more balanced division of services between community care and hospitals; however in practice most expenditure was on the hospitals (DHSS/Welsh Office 1971). At the same time a pressure group, the Campaign for the Mentally Handicapped, was set up by concerned individuals receiving a grant from the DHSS. It aimed to promote the welfare of the handicapped through training activities, research, and a campaign for better services.

Two years later, Townsend (1973) analysed the failure of community care policies to root firmly into the system of caring for the handicapped. First, he considered that two fundamentally contradictory policies had been pursued, namely of trying to reduce the role of hospitals, whilst at the same time allocating them more funds and status as a response to the findings of ill-treatment and lack of resources at Ely Hospital. Second, the power and control held by the Secretary of State over local authority care provision was weak, because of the system of care and the length of the administrative chain. Third, the medical and nursing professions called for better resources and an end to negative criticism as the proposed changes in policy threatened their existence. The final part of his analysis regarded as a political act the use of large institutions to isolate the mentally handicapped within a paternalistic and oppressive setting, with few alternative provisions for care or treatment, or alternative channels of complaint. Community care policies did not, then, take off at this juncture, despite an expressed commitment to it by the government.

Meanwhile, the Education Act 1970 had brought severely handicapped children into its scope in schools for the educationally subnormal (severe). In 1968 the Hester Adrian Centre for the Study of Learning Processes had been established at Manchester University, with Peter Mittler as director. In 1973, Mittler was made the first Professor of Special Education. In 1972, the Report of the Committee on Nursing recommended a new structure for the training of nurses and a new breed of 'care-staff' to care for mentally handicapped children and adults (DHSS 1972a).

The Children Act 1975 enshrined attitude changes towards the rights and needs of all children, with the welfare of the child being put first in both adoption and care cases. That handicapped children needed to be treated as far as possible like non-handicapped children was part of the newly developing attitudes. In 1975, the National Development Group for the Mentally Handicapped was set up under the chairmanship of

Professor Peter Mittler. This group, although disbanded in 1980, worked at a central government level to commit adequate resources to the needs of the mentally handicapped and to achieve a unified organizational commitment throughout the country. Section 10 of the Education Act 1976 laid down that in future, handicapped children should be educated in ordinary, not special, schools, except where this was impracticable or incompatible with the efficiency of the school or would involve unreasonable public expenditure. These new attitudes of greater community care were also a main focus of the Report of the Committee on Child Health Services (DHSS 1976b) which proposed an integrated child health service to cover handicapped as well as non-handicapped children, including district handicap teams. These proposals reinforced those of the Sheldon Report (Ministry of Health 1967) which had recommended the increase in provision of multi-disciplinary assessment centres for young handicapped children. Prior to this, a hospital paediatric outpatient clinic was followed by referral to other specialists, a frequently exhausting and time-consuming system for parents, which often resulted in conflicting advice being given and a fully comprehensive assessment never being undertaken.

This gradual moving towards community care received added impetus from Oswin (1978) in a study of children living in the special care wards of eight mental handicap hospitals. After describing the shortcomings of the hospitals, the problems facing the nursing staff and their lack of support from the medical profession and the public, she put forward a number of radical suggestions to improve the situation of the hospitalized children, whilst recognizing that integrating them into the community should be the overall aim.

During the 1970s more research data was being produced regarding residential care and the differential effects of certain types of residential institution. As director of the Wessex Regional Health Authority's Health Care Evaluation Team, Kushlick (1970) has had a significant influence on policy and practice. Since the 1960s his team had been doing very detailed evaluation and monitoring of traditional hospital-based services. Their data has pointed to the failure of these services to provide a satisfactory environment for handicapped people. On the basis of this, small locally-based units with a more domestic, homelike form of care have been set up as an alternative to hospitals. Further developments have been the construction of detailed guidelines for day-to-day running of the residential establishments. All this work, which mainly uses behavioural approaches, is still the subject of evaluation.

The differential approaches to residential care were the subject of a study by King, Raynes, and Tizard (1971) which investigated the administrative processes, staffing, patterns of care, and child management techniques in a hundred separate living units in twenty-six different establishments for mentally handicapped children. Two major types of management structure were identified. Although no measurable evidence was available to indicate that the child-oriented management practices of some institutions were better than the institutionally oriented practices of others, current values and beliefs would indicate that the former is the preferred type of management practice.

In the USA, work has also been undertaken to assess the effects of differing institutional climates on the mentally handicapped (Butterfield and Zigler 1968). Klaber (Butterfield and Baumeister 1970:165) sums up recent research conclusions regarding institutional rearing as:

'1. Institutional child-rearing is generally less conducive to child growth and development than normal home care; and

2. Some institutional environments are less harmful to child growth and development than others.'

Just after these findings were emerging about the differing effects of institutional management practices two significant reports were produced about the educational and nursing needs of the handicapped. The Warnock Report (DES 1978) proposed the extension of the concept of special educational need to cover one in five of the school population. It recommended the abolition of statutory categories of handicap but the retention of special schools for some children, including boarding schools. A year later, the Jay Report (DHSS 1979a) proposed a common training for staff working in health and social services facilities, leading to a Certificate in Social Service. It also proposed a model of care that would ensure that all mentally handicapped people, whatever their degree of handicap, could get the residential and other services they needed within a generic framework and in their own locality.

The two decades prior to 1980 saw considerable changes in public attitudes towards the young handicapped, with them beginning to be treated more like non-handicapped children, and the concept of community care taking a firmer hold. These changes in attitude and policy were expressed in the number of children in long-stay hospitals. In 1970 there were 6,093 (DHSS 1972b) severely mentally handicapped children under fifteen years of age in such hospitals, whilst in 1974 the number was estimated at approximately 4,500 (DHSS 1977). This slow decline has continued, albeit in a hesitant and long-drawn-out manner.

CURRENT PROVISION AND DEVELOPMENTS FOR
HANDICAPPED CHILDREN

On entering the 1980s the community care concept is to the fore-front, with children rarely, if ever, being admitted to mental deficiency hospitals on a long-stay basis. The district handicap teams as proposed by the Court Report (DHSS 1976b) are part of an integrated health service and multi-disciplinary assessment centres for young handicapped children and are part of the National Health Service provisions, particularly in large centres of population. However, despite advances proposed by the Education Act 1976, many children continue to be educated in special schools, some of which require boarding. The generic Social Services Departments are now responsible for day centres for the handicapped and supportive services for them and their families.

Although handicapped children are now catered for mainly within the community, circumstances may occur in the life of any child that necessitate a stay, however brief, in residential care. Many of the reasons for admission will be similar to those for the non-handicapped, although there is the probability that such reasons will occur more frequently for the handicapped as a result of the additional strain that a handicapping condition imposes on the child, his family, and environment.

Recently much has been written about the effect of different handicapping conditions on the child and his family and the considerable burden borne by his parents in caring for him (Hewett 1970; Gath 1978; Kirman 1972; Burton 1974; Woodburn 1975; Gregory 1976; Kew 1976; Wilkin 1979). From these and the numerous other works recently published, three common findings stand out. First, a handicapping condition can impose a severe burden and strain on the child and his family; second, families frequently do have the abilities (albeit latent) to care for their child even if he is severely handicapped; and third, and perhaps most significantly, to enable them to cope they must be provided with readily available information, emotional support, and practical assistance right from the time of handicap being suspected, be it at birth or later.

These findings have been fully reinforced by the recent books written by parents of handicapped children. Some of these have described only their personal experiences, whilst others have collated those of a group of parents (Park 1967; Wilks and Wilks 1974; Hannam 1975). Fox (1974) presented transcripts of interviews with parents of handicapped children. Although a member of the medical profession, he undertook the interviews informally as a non-professional lay-man. His study focused on parents' attitudes to services they have received, as did a study of Scottish families with a young cerebral palsied child (Tarran 1981).

Since the mid-1970s a number of self-help books for parents and professionals have been published (Collins and Collins 1975; Jeffree and McConkey 1977; Stone and Taylor 1977; Russell 1978). Several books giving guidance on suitable toys for specific handicaps were produced by the Toy Libraries Association (1975) which had been recently formed. At the same time several children's books were written to cater for the handicapped child and his siblings (Fanshawe 1975; Larsen 1976).

All these books gave a considerable boost to the status of and service provision for handicapped children, focusing on a policy of community care. Parents were being encouraged, wherever possible, to care for their child at home, giving him as normal a life as possible, yet bearing in mind the needs of the whole family.

A contributing factor to community care has been the concept of 'normalization'. Although in common use in Scandinavia, it has not rooted so firmly in Britain and interpretations of it have been very variable. The basic idea is that the norms, patterns, and conditions of everyday life in the mainstream of society should be made available as nearly as possible to the mentally retarded as their capacity to adjust to society is purely qualitative and even the most severely handicapped person can be 'normalized' in one or more respects. Gunzberg (1970) has been one of the principal exponents of this concept in Britain.

The 1970s also saw the development of a range of new initiatives to assist the handicapped child and his family. The Hester Adrian Research Centre at the University of Manchester has encouraged close collaboration between professionals and parents in the teaching of handicapped children. The Chorley Project, run by Barnardo's NW Division has provided a toy library, a summer play scheme, holiday and short-term care, as well as initiating a professional fostering scheme for hard to place children. Meanwhile, Northgate Hospital in Northumberland has been running a 'Substitute Families Scheme' using non-handicapped families to provide periods of relief for children normally cared for by their parents. A number of similar initiatives have been developed elsewhere, some being of a purely service nature, whilst others have included rigorous evaluation by researchers.

The Portage Project from Wisconsin, USA has been replicated in the Wessex Regional Health Authority as part of the work being undertaken by Dr A. Kushlick and his team. In this project, community workers are given intensive structured training for one week. They then undertake precision-teaching of skills to parents to enable them to teach their own handicapped child relevant skills. Home visitors are supervised by an educational psychologist with no previous experience of this form of precision-teaching. As a move beyond the replication, the Wessex Portage Project has focused on the teachers and the monitoring system.

A strongly community care oriented initiative is NIMROD, set up in South Glamorgan in 1979 as a joint venture between the Welsh Office and the health and local authorities. Its aim is to promote the health, safety, and human rights of each handicapped client, helping each one to live as normally as possible. The service is to be fully documented.

Despite the numerous developments as mentioned above, some children remain in long-stay hospitals. A recently established pressure group, EXODUS, has recently called for a clear programme culminating in the setting up of sufficient units of care by 1984 so that all children's wards can then be closed. EXODUS, the British Association of Social Workers, and the National Association for Mental Health (MIND) have expressed disquiet about repeated delays by the government in issuing its long-awaited Green Paper on proposals to transfer funds from regional health authorities to local authorities for setting up new small units for long-stay mental handicap patients under nineteen years of age. It is hoped that this Green Paper and the recently formed Jay Action Group will help to realize the aspirations of the previous decade to develop community care to its fullest.

THE NEEDS OF HANDICAPPED CHILDREN AND THEIR FAMILIES AND REASONS FOR ADMISSION TO CARE

Despite the growing emphasis on community care, there will always be some occasions when a period of residence, either in a hospital, children's home, special boarding school, or other placement away from home is necessary. This should now, however, be viewed in the context of the child's whole life and environment, with the firm expectation of discharge once the reason for admission has been fulfilled. As a result the needs of the child and his family on discharge from residential care are an integral part of their whole needs and problems.

On the basis of this discussion of literature and developments in caring for the handicapped, the needs common to all handicapped families, from the time of first suspecting the existence of a handicapping condition, can be spelt out. Briefly these are:

(1) early and continuing information regarding the diagnosis and its prognosis;

(2) practical assistance with daily management problems, either by admission to a day placement or retention of the child at home, according to the needs of the individual family;

(3) home-visits from a trained person who can give assistance with the practical and emotional problems of the family;

(4) facilities to encourage contact between parents of handicapped children, especially for purposes of mutual support; including the availability of suitable helpful literature at a level that can be understood by parents of widely varying abilities;

(5) facilities to provide substitute care for the child in order to give parents and siblings times for rest and for undertaking occasional activities in which it is impossible to include the handicapped child; holiday provision for both parents and child is important, either together or separately; and

(6) educational provision, whenever possible, within the normal school system.

Given that these needs are fulfilled, parents will be enabled to care for their child at home in a way that minimizes the need for residential care for whatever reason. As a result, reasons for admission are likely to be for quite specific needs such as hospitalization for purposes of investigation, treatment, specific operations, or perhaps illness. After these it is probable that the child will be discharged directly to home. Substitute care in children's homes may provide relief for parents, either on a short-term holiday basis for a number of weeks or for a longer stay should family circumstances prevent the parents from continuing to care for their child. Examples of such admissions would be to allow parents to take siblings on a special holiday where it would be impossible to include the handicapped child, or simply to give the parents a holiday. Equally, particularly if the children's home is geared up to providing holidays, such provision may be the best way of providing the child with the experience of a holiday away from his parents and home as one of the first steps towards encouraging his independence. Sometimes family circumstances independent of the handicapped child, such as the illness of a parent, the birth of another child, or the death of a family member, may also require a period of admission to residential care. However, since the style of management of the residential establishment can have a significant effect on the mental development and psychological well-being of the child, as discussed earlier, it is important that a suitable establishment is chosen, however short the intended period of residence. A period of residence with foster parents or a substitute family may be used as an alternative to a stay in a children's home; in some areas special schemes have been developed such as the above-mentioned Substitute Family Scheme by Northgate Hospital in Northumberland. Such schemes go far towards minimizing the potentially upsetting experience of a period in residential care by not only enabling the child to feel comfortable in familiar surroundings, but by encouraging stays to be of a frequency that will prevent the build-up of stress in parents.

These above-mentioned situations are the most frequent reasons for a child's admission to residential care. It should not, however, be forgotten that since the concept of community care has been more widely accepted, attempts are being made to empty the children's wards of mental deficiency hospitals. This policy is resulting in the discharge into the community of severely multiply handicapped children of school age who were admitted to hospitals before community care practices were so seriously considered. For these children, who are now perhaps teenagers, the problems of being discharged from care are much more difficult. However, they may be fewer in number than the younger children who experience residential care as part of a continuum of care. The needs of these two groups will be considered together as the difference is likely to be one of severity rather than type, so the same principles of good social work practice can be applied to work with both groups.

THE EXPERIENCE OF LEAVING RESIDENTIAL CARE

Chapter 1 has outlined the process of departure from residential care, presenting five distinct phases, namely (1) planning, (2) review, (3) preparation, (4) departure, and (5) after-care. For the handicapped child leaving care these five phases will now be considered in relation to the concepts of continuity and change, decision-making, and planning, three concepts discussed earlier. The needs of the child and his family will be examined to see how best the social worker can assist them through the five phases involved in the departure process.

As the eventual return to the community should be the ultimate goal of planning for admission to care, then the residential stay should be part of the continuum of care rather than a separate entity. Righton (1973) was a particular advocate of this approach. The concept of continuity in the care process is assisted by the principles behind the unitary approach to social work practice. The original exponents of this method of practice wrote 'Our definition of social work practice focuses on the linkages and interactions between people and resource systems and the problems to be faced in the functioning of both individuals and systems' (Pincus and Minahan, in Specht and Vickery 1977:78). Seven main functions were seen as part of the social work task. In each of the processes of discharge the appropriate functions will be considered.

The stages prior to admission will involve the perception of a problem, such as the first suspicions of handicap in a young child or the initial signs that parents are feeling unable to cope with the present circumstances of caring for their child and need a break. A tell-tale sign may be that the child looks less well cared for than usual. Similarly, bouts of crying or excessive irritability in the mother may indicate that she is under more strain than usual. For a child in long-term residential care, who had been admitted without plans for eventual discharge, the problem may be indicated, not by signs from the child, but instead by changes in hospital policy reflecting the changing views of society towards the long-term hospitalization of handicapped children. Once the problem has been perceived a full investigation and analysis of the situation will be required in order to make decisions about how best to meet the needs of the child and his family. Such an assessment might take place in out-patient visits to an Assessment Centre, where investigations regarding the suspected handicap can be undertaken by members of the District Handicap Team. For the mother showing signs of strain, discussions with a social worker can help clarify her feelings and problems. Decisions can be taken about how best to meet her needs and plans can be made to achieve these goals, perhaps by arranging a short holiday for the child in a home specially catering for holidays for the handicapped or with a substitute family. For the child in a long-stay hospital a multi-disciplinary team may focus its energies on deciding how best the ultimate goal of discharge can eventually be achieved given the resources available locally. Here the social worker's function may be to contribute to the development of policy and the highlighting of unmet needs. Plans can be made regarding how best the policy can be put into practice and how additional resources could be created to fulfil unmet needs. This may be by developing suitable foster-care schemes or perhaps small group houses within the community.

Admission to residential care and/or maintenance within it will be the next stages within the process. It is at this time that parents and child will gain the bulk of their experience of residential care, but the stages preceding and following it will also be significant. The experience of discharge will thus be dependent not only on the experience of being in care, but also on the planning that has been undertaken prior to admission.

In the planning stage the parents and child should be closely involved; a particular social work function should be to help parents to enhance and use effectively their own problem-solving and coping capacities. The social worker can do this by enabling them to discuss their own situation, needs, and resources in the light of the problem they are facing and the alternative solutions that are available. Information and guidance will be required on a variety of topics, depending on whether the admission is for medical, educational, or social purposes. Here the social worker will need to establish links between the child and his family and the resource systems to be used such as school, hospital, or holiday home. In the case of a handicapped child being ill-treated by his parents, the social worker's function will be to act as an agent of social control whilst behaving in as therapeutic a manner as possible for both child and family.

Whatever the purpose of the admission, the field social worker should be one of the main actors in the decision-making process as she is in a position to evaluate the risks and the potential losses and gains involved in the admission. She will be able to act as an advocate for the family whilst understanding the medical, educational, or social needs, implications, and resources for admission and after-care. For the residential worker this period will be important in enabling her to understand the child, and his problems and needs in the wider context of his total situation, thus ensuring some continuity in his experience despite a change in physical environment.

During the residential period the child will experience the provisions made for him in a variety of ways, depending on the purposes of the admission. The child at risk of physical or emotional harm from his parents will experience a sense of protection; the child who has been admitted to care for a short stay in order to initiate a behaviour modification programme or a particular form of treatment may experience a controlling or enabling element; and enablement, albeit delayed since the effects are not immediately felt, may be the experience of a child admitted for a surgical operation. An essential function of this period is the reviewing of the original plans, the goals set and how nearly these have been achieved. By keeping a continual check on progress and making any minor alterations to means or goals, the maximum benefit can be obtained from the time spent in care. If necessary, alternative means can be used to achieve the set goals. Throughout this a frank and informed dialogue is required between all parties involved. It is likely that the residential worker or hospital staff will have more immediate knowledge of the impact of the experience of residential care on the child and is therefore in a position well suited to judge his vulnerability to risk, should significant changes be made in his programme. Equally, the field social worker can represent the reality of the situation to which it is planned the child should return. For both social workers, their function at this time will be to facilitate interaction and modify and build relationships between people within resource systems, for example by working with parents to reduce marital tensions or strains imposed by caring for their child. It might be possible to initiate support from friends, family, or neighbours, thus reducing burdens on the parents. Within the residential care setting relationships between staff might require attention in order to best meet the needs of the child.

During this review period, when decisions have to be made about alternative courses of further action, the concepts of choice and the associated elements of risk are ones that will figure quite strongly. Given that there is more than one course of action available (hence the need for review), the advantages and disadvantages of two or more possibilities have to be weighed up and the risks attached to each, assessed. This can be particularly difficult when elements of both courses are unknown, thus indicating an unknown outcome. In such situations, the greater the knowledge and experience of the various participants the fewer unknowns there will be, but given the individual nature of each child and situation the outcome can never be fully known. Even if the same child has been in the same situation before, the passage of time and the previous experience will immediately contribute two new variables.

Having made a decision and chosen one course of action, namely that of the child being discharged from residential care, other factors may still remain undecided, for example at what point in his treatment, education, or general state should he be discharged, to where and to whom. Some of these factors will have been decided at the review stage, whilst others will require the examination of alternatives, realistic choices, and the eventual making of decisions in the preparation stage. It is important that, even though some decisions have been made for changes in the child's life, an element of continuity is maintained in order to prevent a total disruption to his life-style and emotional attachments. The preparation stage is of great importance, then, not only for the purposes of organizing the practical details of his departure and ensuing life, but also to help him begin to make the necessary emotional adjustments. During this time the impending sense of loss will be anticipated, as will the expectations of new or resumed relationships. The amount of emotional preparation required is likely to bear a relation to the impact of the residential experience on the child in both emotional and practical terms; the length of stay and whether or not it has been enjoyable; the amount of contact he has been able to maintain with his family and friends outside; and the problems that are solved during or anticipated after his stay. Both the field and residential social worker have important roles to play in the preparation phase, although it is difficult to spell out who should do which tasks. The unitary approach to social work practice advocates that workers in all settings should possess the same skills, although the actual tasks on which they use them may vary. Introducing a child to a new day care centre or foster family or re-establishing relationships between him and his family may be important tasks in the preparation phase. Enabling visits of the family, by assisting with transport, will be as valid a task as teaching him new skills or talking with him about experiences during his stay. Sometimes the planning for his needs on discharge will be as important as other more immediate practical tasks or emotional preparation. Examples are making plans for travel home, visits back to the residential centre, the provision of aids and adaptations necessary for his care at home, or support groups for his parents. In some cases a behaviour modification programme might be embarked upon to change aspects of the child's behaviour that his parents or others find difficult or disturbing to deal with. Parents, too, might need to be warned about the possible effects of residence on the child's behaviour once he is discharged home. Attention-seeking or changed patterns of behaviour can be disturbing to parents who may try to compensate for their child's absence from home by treatment that exacerbates his changed and difficult behaviour.

By the end of the preparation phase, both the child and those around him should have as clear an idea as possible of the practical details surrounding his actual departure and life in the ensuing months. Emotional preparation should have encouraged the loosening of some and strengthening of other emotional ties, whilst recognizing that even despite these changes the actual moment of departure will present new dimensions of emotional experience that cannot be anticipated.

The day of departure, which may have been anticipated with feelings of dread or longing, may turn out to be an anticlimax for the child. This is less likely to happen if good planning and preparation has been undertaken beforehand and the actual process of departure occurs without hitch. At this point it is particularly helpful to preserve the feelings of continuity in the child's life by planning for a return visit, letter, or telephone call to the residential centre. This task can be useful for all participants; for the child it can allow him to retain some emotional contact with care-staff and other residents with whom he has spent a meaningful part of his life; the staff will appreciate knowing how the young child is faring now he is no longer in their care and for parents the maintenance of contact can be particularly helpful for resolving practical or emotional problems that are being experienced once the child is home. The residential centre may also be the provider of long-term support services that enable the child to be cared for in the community, such as short-stay holidays or day-relief for parents, or for information and resources. In some situations the feeling of need to maintain such contacts will be minimal, for example when the admission was for short-term holiday purposes. In others, such as the child being discharged to specially recruited foster-parents after some years in a hospital, the need for continued contact for emotional and practical support may be high.

The point of discharge is always likely to contain some elements of risk as the plans made earlier are put into practice. Not only may some of the most carefully laid plans go astray, but the emotional reactions of participants cannot always be anticipated. By encouraging flexible attitudes and discussing possible alternative arrangements, the negative effects of any necessary last-minute changes to plans can be minimized.

At the time of discharge from residential care, residential and field social workers may have similar functions with regard to the dispensing of material resources such as new clothes, travel facilities, and aids and equipment. It may be that some of these tasks can be dealt with during the preparation phase, but for the child going to a new home or one from which he has been long absent, the introduction to new pieces of equipment or changes in the environment is important. Care must be paid to the way in which the introduction is undertaken, not only so that technical information and demonstrations of equipment are made clear for parents and child, but with regard to its emotional significance. The child coming home with legs in plaster after a surgical operation will react very differently, to his bed being moved downstairs out of his own bedroom, from the child who moves in to his own bedroom in a new foster-home after many years of sharing bedrooms in a children's home.

The field social worker can contribute to the settling in of a child returning to or moving into the community by facilitating interaction and helping to build relationships between the family members as they undertake the new tasks of living together. The child returning home after a holiday will respond very differently from a child who is embarking on a new life-style. At this stage social workers should be aware of the way in which the agency's policies and practice relating to the day of departure affect the individuals concerned. It may be possible to identify needs or gaps in resources and thus contribute to new policy to help overcome the dysfunctional aspects. For example, parents travelling a long distance to collect their child whom they have been unable to see very regularly may find that it is easier in practical and emotional terms, and a greater sense of continuity is preserved, if they can stay overnight before taking the child home.

It is at the point of departure or shortly afterwards that community support and services will become important to the child and his family in enabling them to live together in as happy and healthy a way as possible. The field social worker can help to establish and encourage links between the family and the various resource systems that are available in the community, for example, a toy library, a parents' group, special educational facilities, or a holiday play-scheme. Links between the family and its own informal support network should also be encouraged and given support wherever possible. The process of after-care, which takes place once the child is home, can have very different meanings according to the purpose of the admission. After an admission to hospital for medical purposes, prescribed after-care may be the attendance at out-patient medical clinics for some months to assess the success of the treatment. In such cases, social after-care is also likely to be necessary as the child may be exhibiting behaviour disturbances since discharge, thus requiring some help through behaviour modification, or, more simply, he and his parents may appreciate the continued concern shown in their welfare by a representative of the residential agency. The exchange of letters, photographs, and visits should be part of the after-care process. Sometimes plans need to be made for further spells of residential care and this too can be part of the after-care stage.

For a child with new foster-parents, adapting to life in the community may present particular threats as both will suddenly be faced with many new experiences and situations for which their previous experiences may not be adequate preparation. The feelings of continuity and security represented by return visits to the residential agency or by home-visits from its social worker may help both child and family cope more adequately with the new situations.

Ambivalence may be felt if the after-care services remind the child or his family of an experience they found difficult and would prefer to forget. In all situations, the family and the social worker will need to decide between them the point at which further after-care is no longer required for practical or emotional reasons. In some cases, the after-care may, however, be in the form of continuing support from the residential agency, if this is the way in which local services for the handicapped are organized. For example, children discharged from a long-stay hospital to a small group home in the community may be provided with long-term practical and emotional support services from the hospital that may be acting as the local resource centre. This situation is particularly likely to occur whilst services based on community care concepts are still being developed. Hopefully the time is not far away when all handicapped children will be catered for in the community so that the only hospital after-care or support services required will be those that follow a period of hospitalization for purely medical reasons.

DISCUSSION

The last two decades have seen significant changes in policy relating to the care of the handicapped child and his family. In the early 1950s when consideration was being given to the effects of institutionalization on handicapped children, Kirman (1951:531) wrote 'a decision to place a child in an institution on account of mental deficiency is almost never in the child's interests, but it may be in the interests of another child or in that of the parents themselves.' By the late 1970s community care policies for all client groups were to the forefront and were being exhibited by planning, practice, and research initiatives, for example the Kent Community Care Project for the frail elderly (Challis and Davies 1980).

Given these changes in policy, current practice is to try to cater for all the needs of even the most severely handicapped child within the community, so that admission to long-stay hospitals is a practice of the past. Hand in hand with this is the discharge of all children currently in long-stay hospitals to homes in the community, to small group homes run by the health or social services, to specially recruited foster-families, or to the child's own parents. Any periods of residential care in the life of a handicapped child should be as part of a continuum of care in the community. Whether the admission is for medical, educational, or social reasons, the eventual return to the community should be the ultimate goal, planned for prior to admission, even though the details of the discharge from care may be hazy at that stage.

Once admitted, the five distinct phases involved in the process of discharge will all play a significant part in ensuring that the transition from life in a residential setting to living within the community causes the least negative long-term effects on the child and his family or care-givers. Even a very short period of residence can be traumatic if badly managed, when the family and child are already under the additional strains imposed by living with a handicapping condition. For a child whose memory recalls nothing other than life in a long-stay institution, leaving residential care may be even more disruptive. The effects on residential care staff can also be significant when they have devoted long hours to the intimate care of a severely handicapped child. For these reasons, as well as for the impact on the informal support givers and the local community, the process of helping the child on leaving residential care requires very sensitive and carefully thought out social work practice, combined with close collaboration and liaison with other professionals such as health visitors, teachers, and general practitioners who are likely to be equally closely involved with the child and family.

5   The Elderly   *Paul Brearley*

This chapter will extend a discussion which began in our earlier book (Brearley *et al*. 1980:ch. 7) and should be read in conjunction with that chapter. It will therefore not deal in detail with a number of issues which are of direct relevance, although it is intended to be complete in itself.

ON OPTIMISM . . .

In recent years it has been increasingly recognized that ageing and old age are important areas for study and research and for social work practice. The range and quality of literature and practice in the field have improved substantially and it no longer seems a forlorn hope that at least some older people will be helped to return to live in their own homes after a period in residential care. Certainly a substantial number of people now stay in old people's homes for planned short periods for a variety of reasons and expect to, and do, return home. Similarly many older people are admitted to hospital for treatment and rehabilitation and expect to return to their previous living situation. Although it might once have been argued with some truth that few older people who entered the institutional system would ever leave, except after their death, the picture is no longer so clear-cut. It is, therefore, important and relevant to review some of the issues which arise in helping older people to leave institutions.

. . . AND REALISM

It should be remembered, however, that people entering residential care are likely to be very old and frail. For many of these people it would be unrealistic and probably unfair that they should be admitted with any expectation of being able to return to independent living within the current range of services. Although researchers have noted for many years the apparently quite high proportions in old people's homes who have a reasonable level of self-care abilities there have been few practical responses. Social work with older people continues to be undervalued and to be regarded in many areas as less important than other forms of social work. Further, the current financial climate hardly provides a basis for an optimistic view of the provision of resources necessary to give support to those older people who do want to return to independent life.

Before proceeding to discuss ways of helping people to leave institutional care, some consideration of available services is necessary to provide a background for detailed discussion. Jones (1980) offers a basic classification of social services which provides a useful starting point. She identifies, first, personal social services in Social Services Departments: these include casework techniques, advice services, befriending services, domiciliary services, and individual protection schemes. Second, group support services, including social clubs and day care. Third, she lists total care services, the main form of which, in Social Services Departments, is residential care. It would not be appropriate to review here the entire range of services provided by local authorities but a number of basic points can be made.

It is clear that services as a whole fall short of the total need, although such a comment must be seen against the background of current norms and expectations. As Bebbington (1978) has shown from a review of three major surveys of older people conducted between 1962 and 1976, considerable strides have been made in provision. There is evidence that the proportions of people receiving help at home have increased markedly yet it is even more true now than it was in the early 1960s that 'the old and the socially isolated are those who receive services' (Bebbington 1978:8). The increase in the number of very elderly — and therefore the increase in isolation and incapacity — has reduced the real gains. A second important factor is the current inadequacy and ineptness of assessment approaches in allocating services to individuals. As the BASW Special Interest Group on Ageing have put it, for example, 'The Meals on Wheels Service illustrates the current, all too frequent, practice of not making a proper assessment of an individual's real need. The result is that services can be wasteful and ineffective' (BASW 1978:18). Third, the community services remain unevenly distributed. In some authorities up to 10–15 per cent of all older people receive home helps during a year whilst in other areas the total is 5 per cent or less. Similarly Bosanquet (1978) reports eightfold differences between authorities in the London area in the amount spent on meals. This may partly represent real differences in need: older people congregated, for example, in deprived inner city areas are likely to make heavier demands. However this does not account for the whole picture: to take an alternative example, many of the coastal retirement areas have lower levels of home help service. In areas with larger proportions of older people there are relatively fewer younger people to provide services.

One further point is important. Need is both objectively and subjectively defined and met. Many studies confirm that the expression of demand for service and the assessment of need seems to depend at least to some extent on the attitudes and beliefs of the individuals involved. Although attempts to develop more systematic and objective measures for allocating services are necessary to the overall use and development and provision, such attempts must also be seen in the light of subjective factors.

This chapter will be concerned to set out the broad context within which realistic help can be given to older people who wish to move from institutional care back to what is usually called community living. It will explore some of the issues which arise from innovations in services, the flexible use of existing provision, and the role of informal care, as well as consider the importance of individual rights in a formal and complex system of provisions. On this basis there will be discussion of assessment of and practical help for individuals who leave care.

WHAT CAN BE DONE WITH SERVICES?

Social services have been described as providing alternatives for older people in a number of different ways. One commonly used term is the 'continuum of care'. In one sense this may be used to mean that services provide as broad a range of facilities as possible. The individual is expected to be able to move freely within the total range of resources and to be at the right place at the right time for his own special needs. One view of this regards the continuum as a process of growing dependence. The older person outside the caring system is fully independent and as his needs increase so he moves into and through the system and becomes increasingly dependent until he reaches a stage of total care. There is evidence that some people in institutional care have been through such a process of increasing dependence on services, but the evidence that the caring system can be seen in such rational and precise terms is very sparse indeed. An alternative view of the caring continuum stresses the importance of a circularity of movement in which the client or patient is seen as entering forms of service in which he will receive treatment, care, and rehabilitation and eventually be returned to his original situation. This view would, for instance, see the task of hospitals as being to return older people to their homes as soon as possible, perhaps after a transitional stay in a nursing home or other residential home. In fact there does seem to be considerable evidence that many older people are wrongly placed in institutions and in the community and many of them do appear to get stuck in the various parts of the system. Again, then, there is limited evidence that people move freely along any form of continuum and there is considerable evidence to the contrary.

A slightly different but closely related view stresses the importance of choice as a principle for policy and practice. It is argued that there should be a range of provisions and a set of strategies for making a variety of options available to older people so that they can choose for themselves the kind of old age that they want. This assumption that the main forms of services do serve as options has been effectively challenged.

Plank (1977) has argued that 'it is very doubtful whether in practice domiciliary care in private households, sheltered housing and old people's homes do act as options for individual old people in need of help and support' (p. 5). In the first place the options do not always exist and in the second place the cost of providing care at home equivalent to that available in residential homes is considerable. Furthermore such care is not often available. Real choice involves offering at least two possibilities of available services, each of which will offer a comparable level of care. With one or two innovative exceptions services which are substitutable in this sense have not been available and they therefore do not represent alternatives.

A further issue is the underlying assumption in discussions of choice and substitutability of services that need is a constant factor, that different approaches can be used to meet the same needs with equal effect. Need is both an objective and a subjective phenomenon and it seems likely that two people with objectively similar needs will make different choices about services. It also seems likely that given a choice between, for example, full care in a residential home and an equivalent level of care in their own home, most people will choose the latter.

Services do not therefore act as alternatives either in the sense that older people can move freely within the caring system according to their needs or in the sense that services provide equivalent levels of care. This does not, however, negate the desirability of creating options for older people. It may be that to remain at home or to return home carries the risk of reduced and less adequate service, but the right to take that risk to preserve a sense of self-direction and control over his life may be more important to an older person than the security offered by residential care.

The discussion of choice in service provision has developed primarily around the residential care/community care division. Since the 1950s one of the dominant themes in discussions of policy and provision has been the advocacy of community care and the denigration of residential care. In his important study Townsend (1962) argued very strongly that services should be developed to make it possible for the older person to live in the community actively and independently and that residential homes should be replaced by sheltered forms of housing. Almost twenty years later the Disability Alliance, in a report drafted principally by Townsend, argued that 'once there is a substantial amount of well-designed sheltered housing within each local community, and once there is sufficient social service support for families and for the isolated elderly, we see little cause for the continued existence of residential homes' (Disability Alliance 1979:42).

One underlying assumption of the advocacy of alternatives to residential care is that such care is damaging to those who experience it. One of the most influential contributions to this view is that of Goffman (1961) who argues that 'total institutions' are characterized by the performance of all aspects of daily life in the same place under the same control, and in the company of others who tend to be treated alike; all phases of the day's activities are tightly scheduled; and all activities are brought together in one plan to fulfil the official aims of the institution. This approach is complemented by the view of 'institutionalization' as an illness characterized by a high degree of dependency, withdrawal, and apathy and caused by elements within the institution (Barton 1959). This negative perspective can be challenged in a number of ways. First, there is reason to believe that the behaviours noted among older people which have been attributed to living in an institutional environment are probably as much attributable to feelings of abandonment and anticipatory loss following making the decision to enter residential care. Withdrawal and apathy are also a feature of the period before admission and it is possible that the institutional environment *per se* is not the cause of negative behaviours although it may contribute to maintaining them (Tobin and Lieberman 1976). A second reason to question the totally negative view of residential care is that many residents seem to be content. Harris (1968) found that most residents are quite content to be living in care and a more recent study of a smaller group of residents found that 60 per cent said they had wanted to become residents, whilst 35 per cent said they had not (Shaw and Walton 1979). Of the residents 73 per cent said they thought it best to stay in the home and the authors of the study said that most people could identify reasons for admission which seemed convincing to themselves. A wish to enter a residential home is not, of course, an indication that the older person is free from stress, or anxiety, nor is it any indication of whether he would have preferred other forms of care given a realistic choice. Some evidence does suggest that older people who want to go into residential care are overwhelmingly in the minority (Reynolds 1980; Foster and Remfry 1981). A further reason to question the negative assumptions about residential care is that there is evidence that the residential environment can be improved to provide a more acceptable quality of life (Brearley 1977; Ward, P. 1980). It may be that it is not so much institutional living which is damaging but impoverished care of any kind (Butler, Oldman, and Wright 1979).

A particularly important aspect of the use of residential care is the argument that many people are misplaced, not only in homes but in hospitals, nursing homes, sheltered housing, and other forms of care. A study of behavioural problems among patients in geriatric and psycho-geriatric wards and residents of homes in Manchester found a considerable overlap between agencies in terms of the types of clients and patients catered for. Residents, for instance, presented fewer problems of physical dependency than patients in hospital but the study still identified many residents who were doubly incontinent, unable to dress themselves, and who required washing and bathing (Wilkin and Jolley 1979). Similarly a study of residential homes in London found that in a third of the homes there were some residents whom the senior staff thought would be more suitable for hospital placement and many of these took up disproportionate amounts of time because of their level of infirmity (DHSS 1979b). A different aspect of this is the apparently large proportion of older people in residential care whose level of self-care capacity measured objectively is much higher than that of many people waiting for admission, or continuing to function in the community. Evidence of such misplacement has been produced consistently for many years (Townsend 1976). However, it has been argued that such findings should be treated with caution. Residents who are relatively independent tend to be either temporary, or were admitted some years earlier when objectives and criteria were different, or were admitted at a time of crisis as a result of self-neglect and who would probably revert to a similar position if returned to their own home (Kay 1980).

One implication of the argument that many people are misplaced is that the care system for older people is not a unified or co-ordinated system but a set of discrete and relatively autonomous parts (Plank 1978a). There is some evidence that admissions to different forms of care are appropriate on the basis of current norms (Alexander and Eldon 1979) and it may be that the problem of misplacement is the result of lack of movement within and between services rather than initial misplacement. The problem may be one of lack of co-operation and co-ordination (see e.g. Booth 1980; DHSS 1979b) of services rather than one of initial usage.

In reviewing the community care/residential care debate, two preliminary points are therefore important. First, residential care is not necessarily as negative an experience as the proponents of community care have sometimes argued. Second, there is reason to assume that rigid definitions of services and administrative boundaries may contribute to some older people finding themselves in the wrong place for their changing or changed needs.

Although community care has usually been presented, in contrast to the predominantly negative view of residential care, as an ideal and even idealized approach, the reality often falls far short of any ideal. One approach to the discussion has considered levels of care available in different forms of service, referring to the quantity and quality of care available. Plank (1977), in a study of older people in London living in various residential and community housing circumstances, found marked variations in the levels of care being received. Those older people living in residential homes were receiving significantly higher levels of care than any other groups studied. Those in sheltered housing were found to be in receipt of higher levels of care than those in private households even though levels of need based on self-care measures were greater in the latter group. The cost of providing services to older people in the community to raise the standard of care available to them to a level comparable with that which exists in the residential home is very high and such levels of care are not usually available (Plank 1977). Community care based on the major forms of service provided by local authorities and health services is only likely to be cheaper than institutional care when there is less of it (Scull 1977).

Some mention should also be made here of sheltered housing. The main advocates of the abandonment of residential care have favoured the development of sheltered housing as an alternative. Townsend and Wedderburn (1965) estimated that 5.1 per cent of older people needed sheltered housing, basing this figure on the proportion of their sample who lived alone, had no children within ten minutes' journey, and who were moderately or severely incapacitated. At that time (1963) 0.6 per cent were actually living in such accommodation. A 1976 survey found that 7.9 per cent of older people were living in some form of special housing. Yet the development of sheltered housing is still strongly advocated and if it has a part to play in meeting the needs of 'those who are both incapacitated and socially isolated, then it has only just begun to meet that need' (Bebbington 1978:14).

There is some confusion about the role of sheltered housing, manifest partly in the differing views of housing and social services authorities. On the one hand sheltered housing is seen as a major alternative to residential care for incapacitated older people. It has been argued, at one extreme, that Category II sheltered housing schemes (as defined by DoE Circular 82/69) which are intended for the less active elderly and which have extra facilities provided, should be transferred to Social Services Departments as an alternative to residential accommodation (James and Bytheway 1978). On the other hand, sheltered housing is seen as a preventive provision for relatively fit older people. Some have argued that sheltered housing is predominantly used for relatively fit older people while some more dependent people receive less support; that there is, in other words, a group of moderately dependent people who fall between the criteria of residential care and sheltered housing and receive nothing (Plank 1978b). Others have identified a supposition that the tenants of sheltered housing and the residents of residential accommodation share similar dependency characteristics (Butler, Oldman, and Wright 1979). The development of what has been described as 'very sheltered housing' may be a recognition of the needs of an intermediate group who are unable to live completely independently in the more usual form of specialist housing but who are not as dependent as most people in residential care. Some recent developments in this field have provided additional services in sheltered housing to meet the needs of such groups (see e.g. Brown 1978).

It is clear from this brief review that the use of practical services is a complex matter and that the issues involved are further complicated when discussion is broadened to include informal caring services. Before discussing the use of practical resources to help people leaving institutional living, four further general issues should be noted:

(1) Innovations

Mention has been made here of the gap between provision and total need, of the inadequacy of methods of measuring total need, and of assessing individual need, and of geographical inequalities in provision. One consequence of such a patchy scenario has been a range of innovative schemes which attempt to fill gaps and to provide a more cost-effective service. Davies (1981), however, stresses the need to retain an overall view of broad policy essentials in the face of piecemeal innovations. A number of collections of information about innovations in services for the elderly are available (see e.g. PSSC 1980; Ferlie 1980) and, as Davies notes, these indicate a substantial minority of Social Services Departments where no innovations have occurred. Davies also notes some broad characteristics of innovations: they tend to be geographically localized; they are seldom specific with regard to target clientele − reflecting vagueness in criteria; and innovation tends not to be part of a coherent logic in responding to the overall needs and pressures in an area (Davies 1981).

One difficulty in proceeding to discuss social work practice, therefore, is that whilst many interesting and apparently useful approaches are available, in *some* areas, few innovations have been sufficiently generalized for it to be possible to include them in a general prescription for action.

(2) Flexibility

Stress has also been put on the importance of flexibility in the creation of individually organized 'packages' of services. Three elements of the need for flexibility in future development seem particularly important. First, there should be a more imaginative use of resources to meet existing need; second, a differential use of resources may help to increase their acceptability to those who reject help in its present form; and third, better information and identification procedures are needed to recognize unmet need and to ensure that older people are aware of their entitlement to resources.

In order to meet these requirements change must take place on many levels. At an individual level all professional and voluntary workers can contribute to meeting both individual and family need by a flexible use of resources – if planning in a local area is sufficiently coherent and co-ordinated to make such flexibility possible. Older people leaving institutional living are likely to need a considerable input and variety of carefully planned and co-ordinated help if they are to survive. The most important principle is to begin with the needs expressed and perceived in the older person's situation and to seek resources to meet these needs: it should not be necessary for the older person to convert his needs into terms that are acceptable to agencies.

(3) Informal Care

At least two distinct issues have been recognized in recent discussions of informal care. First, on the one hand a substantial minority of older people have few social contacts and therefore lack the help and support of other people. Second, it has been argued that the role of the family has become less significant in the provision of care (or what Parker (1981) has called 'tending', the actual work of looking after people who cannot care for themselves), perhaps because the increase in state provision has undermined traditional family provision.

In fact those older people who do have relatives generally receive – and give in return – help and support: people do accept a mutual responsibility. It is those people – particularly the very old – who have no family or close friends to provide care who seem to make greatest demands on the formal care services. The great majority of older applicants for residential care tend to be very old, physically and mentally frail, and socially unsupported. The task of helping such people to return to community living is therefore particularly difficult. The survival of frail older people in the community is very closely bound up with the existence of a supportive network of relatives, friends, and neighbours. Those who go into residential homes tend not to have such a network, and, even if they have, it is often not surprising that families and friends who have carried a heavy burden of care should breathe a sigh of relief at the time of admission and should be reluctant to take up the burden again.

(4) Rights in Danger

In the light of these considerations it is especially important to be aware of the potential for disregarding the rights of the older person, as well as those of the people who provide support. The balancing of rights, and particularly of freedom and protection, is a central concern in work with older people, especially those whose freedom of movement and self-control is curtailed by loss of mobility, changes of accommodation, and consequent dependence. Some general discussion of rights is therefore appropriate.

In 1975 Age Concern England published a brief but significant summary of the most commonly discussed considerations.

The Manifesto lists the following points: Independence, Choice, Self-realization, Income, Health, Accommodation, Occupation, Mobility, and Participation. It emphasizes that all older people should have the freedom to choose their life-style, to have their views heard, to command respect, and to have a continuing influence on events. A document on the rights of old people produced by the National Secular Society (1971) is rather more abstract but stresses similar points. It lists the right to independence, to respect from fellow citizens, to social and financial security, to adequate care and attention, to ample employment opportunities, and the right to creative fulfilment.

Some years ago I listed some of these points in a slightly different form but I see no reason to alter the list. They are identified as rights not so much in the sense that they are morally good but in the sense that some values are necessary if people are to live their lives with basic opportunities for achieving satisfaction. The main elements seem to be:

'(1) choice: opportunities and access to information on which to base choices
'(2) the need to retain independence and individuality
'(3) the right to appropriate accommodation
'(4) dignity and respect: including the right to be different and the right to privacy.'

(Brearley 1977)

It might be tempting to suggest firstly that older people simply have the same rights as everyone else and secondly that they have a right to be protected from the consequences of all the hazards which increasing age can introduce. In relation to the first point it does seem that the needs of older people are different from those of younger people, partly because of the physical changes which the process of ageing brings but mainly because of the dangers created by the social process of ageing. Older people need to establish some rights of protection against society. On the second of these points, although safety is desirable, total security is neither possible nor desirable: risk-taking is a necessary part of life and if people are to choose freely this must involve the right to expose themselves to hazards in the hope of gain.

A further question concerns the primacy of one person's rights over those of another. If an old lady's right to return to her own home can only be maintained by elderly neighbours or by an ageing daughter who is herself unwell some difficult questions arise: do her rights come before the neighbour's right to a peaceful life, or the daughter's right to preserve her own good health? In the case of children, the legal position is clear: the welfare of the child will take precedence. However, the assumption that older people should and can be self-determining inevitably means that their rights must be balanced against those of other adults. A concept of rights involves a corresponding concept of responsibility: if older people have a right to choice then choice must be exercised responsibly. The question of whose rights take precedence is an important one – the answers are neither simple nor straightforward.

An excellent discussion of rights, risk, and older people already exists and there is no need to replicate that discussion here (Norman 1979). Norman's document was intended to encourage discussion of the issues relating to the defence of older people's right of choice. The document should be essential reading for all practitioners working with older people. Several areas of concern are identified: choosing one's home; compulsory care; freedom within residential care; human rights and nursing care; consent to treatment and the right to die; fatal accidents and the role of the coroner's court; and the Court of Protection. One theme of Norman's document, implicitly as much as explicitly, is that the protective services in fact create hazards in special ways as well as reducing them. Not all of the relevant issues can be dealt with here but some of the more obvious examples may serve to illustrate problems.

It has long been recognized that the actions of professional carers introduce changes into the lives of those older people who are least able to bear such changes (Blenkner, Bloom and Nielson 1971). In relation to admission to care Lieberman (1974) points out that although discussion and preparation for the period of transition may be an important contribution to preventing feelings of loss and unhappiness, it may play little part in reducing the risk because such transition involves radical changes and the people admitted to care, for instance, are ill-equipped for the relearning necessary. We should remember, in other words, that the people going into residential care are very frail and dependent and are by definition the least likely to adapt, the least likely to survive, and perhaps the least likely to be able to cope with further change.

This particular example is compounded when related to the practice which still prevails in many areas (Davies 1979) of only allowing patients to be transferred from hospital to residential care in exchange for a resident from the home and vice versa. The system of swapping 'bodies' has its basis in administrative convenience and not in client need, and creates pressures on older people that can only increase the hazards for people already ill-equipped to handle the existing threats to their well-being and adaptations. Similarly the use of compulsory powers to admit to residential care or hospital is likely to compound these problems for the weakest and least well-equipped (Gray 1980b).

Butler and Oldman (1979), in a discussion relating mainly to sheltered housing, outline several ways in which 'people of goodwill' restrict choice and therefore the independence of the older people they are paid to help. They suggest that the lack of sufficient resources makes the concept of choice a fiction for many, and they propose that 'need scales' in local authority resource allocation often neglect to 'measure' both the older person's support network and the influence of his own perception of preferred solutions. Lastly, they propose that the development of a professional mystique emphasizes the power of the professional and the inability of the 'client' to make his own choices.

A final example can be developed directly within the field of institutional provision. It has been well established that institutional living is often related to apathy, institutionalization (Barton 1959; Goffman 1961), and other restrictions on individuals. Whilst many efforts have recently been made to outline good practice (Brocklehurst 1974; Elliott 1975; PSSC

1977) the fact remains that living in institutions involves exposure to risks both during the admission process and within the institution. Before admission takes place it must, therefore, be clear that the risks of such action (which include the likelihood of not being able to return home) are less than those of the current situation.

This brief treatment of a few examples should be enough to illustrate a particularly important point about decision-making and older people. The *safest* course of action may not necessarily be the *best* course; if being safe means giving up the right to self-determination (to return home whatever the dangers) then it may not be acceptable. But this, too, is a simplistic position: an older person's decision to take risks is partly subject to the wishes of those around him to see that he is safe. In reality safety decisions are made on the basis of a complex balancing of competing possibilities.

*   *   *

To summarize the main points established so far, it is obvious that relatively few people who enter residential care are likely to leave for other forms of accommodation: for most it will be their home until they die. A small group of people who are admitted do seem to be capable of returning to alternative and, in some respects, more independent living. Some of these are unable to move because of the lack of suitable alternatives but a few people are able to leave. An increasing number of people are also admitted for short-term care, perhaps to give carers a holiday, or to provide a period of assessment, relief or rehabilitation: sometimes this is only for a week or two but occasionally for several months; sometimes it is a response to urgent need and sometimes on a planned and intermittent basis of 'shared care' to give regular relief to carers. In all these cases a planned and careful approach is clearly relevant. Similarly many older people experience short periods of hospital care and need a planned approach to rehabilitation and after-care. Discussion of planning for leaving care is therefore concerned with two groups: those who enter institutional care expecting to stay but who either do not like it or improve sufficiently to wish to leave;

and those who are admitted to either residential or hospital care expecting to stay for only a limited period and who need some form of help when they leave.

A second major perspective which has been explored is the nature and range of formal and informal resources. It is clear that formal social service provisions are inadequate to meet needs and demands and attempts must be made to develop new forms of service, to use existing resources flexibly, and to interweave an imaginative and flexible package of services to meet individual circumstances. It would be wrong, however, to suggest that it is anything other than difficult and even dangerous for physically and sometimes mentally frail and dependent older people to leave a protected living environment in which they have experienced a high level of care.

Nevertheless safety is not the only consideration: older people have a right to choose their own risks, as long as they can do so responsibly. If they are to choose, however, they need to know the risks they face and this implies a careful assessment and detailed planning.

ASSESSMENT AND PLANNING

Most older people who go into residential care do so because they are no longer able to care for themselves; family strains and loneliness tend to be much less commonly quoted reasons for applications. Two factors seem clear from the existing research. A substantial number of admissions take place urgently as emergencies: one survey, for example, quotes one large county which estimated that 40–50 per cent of admissions presented as emergencies. Second, admissions are closely related to precipitating factors. Pope (1980), for instance, found that in terms of age and medical conditions there was little difference between those admitted as emergencies and those who came in other circumstances. The most important cause of urgent need seems to be the change in circumstances of those who provide support for the older person; but for a smaller group of people admission follows a period of increasing social isolation and deterioration; and for a few it is the result of an unexpected need for a roof over their heads. The importance of the precipitating factor is confirmed in several studies and there is ample evidence that most people in care are physically frail and dependent for basic care on other people. In such circumstances it is probably important to ask why anyone should wish to leave a protected environment which provides a high level of personal care. In fact, as was shown earlier, the majority of older people in homes do seem to be quite content although this must be seen in the light of the tendency of older people to be more accepting of their general circumstances than younger people, wherever they live. It is likely that the expression of contentment or acceptance reflects a realistic awareness of the lack of alternatives rather than any positive preferment of the residential accommodation. It would be inappropriate to advocate a major programme to encourage those who currently live in old peoples' homes to move. This would not only be unrealistic and impossible in view of current resources but those who have given up both the hope or expectation of ever moving, and their home, furniture, and possessions (and therefore the means to move) will inevitably find the idea of change difficult and probably distressing. It is more important to focus attention on planning at the time of application for residential care. If people go in with an expectation that they may make progress and return then this is a very different prospect from being encouraged to leave after giving up all hope of doing so. Yet this, too, has its problems: if everyone admitted to care is encouraged to hope for eventual return home the process of settling in is disrupted. Many hopes will not be fulfilled, which will create discomfort, distress, and disturbance. This inevitably points to the central importance of detailed assessment at the time of admission.

One consequence of the importance of precipitating factors and emergencies is that those with high but less dramatic need are likely to have to wait for some time before admission. It has been argued that people admitted to emergency beds should be discussed as soon as possible and plans for review and possible discharge made (Avon County Council 1980). Clearly it is important to give thorough attention to the needs of older people admitted in haste not only for their own sake but also for the sake of others in need.

Emphasis has also been put on making what is usually called a 'total assessment' of the older person, which involves the collection of information about abilities and the social and physical environment. A decision about what a person can do is concerned not only with basic capacities but also with how those capacities relate to the pressures of the environment. Assessment is also concerned, as was suggested earlier, with the subjective meaning of experiences. Some older people are determined to cope alone in spite of severe difficulties while others will accept high levels of service much sooner: the way people perceive their needs and risks is important. Assessment is therefore about measuring what people can and will do in their environment and relating that to what they wish to do. Some questions will be particularly important, whether in relation to people wanting to enter or to leave institutional living.

(1) What can people do?

There are two ways of approaching the measurement of the capacities of older people. One way is to measure the individual's abilities, focusing on physical and intellectual performance. The second approach, which may be referred to as measuring dependency emphasizes incapacities, measuring the things a person can not do rather than what he can do. It has been argued that in assessing effective health, functional capacity is more important than the presence of disease (Williams 1979). In this view what is important is the ability of the individual to perform those tasks that are essential to everyday living. This can be extended to three broad categories of behaviours which have been helpfully listed by Miller (1979):

(1) Self-care behaviours: habits related to daily functions (eating, sleeping, toileting, self-grooming, and health behaviours).
(2) Task-behaviours: management of tasks assigned because of membership of certain social groups.

(3) Relationship behaviours: interacting with adults including age peers, adult children, adults in authority, and younger associates.

This begins to shift the emphasis away from physical and mental capacities to recognizing the additional importance of the ability to manage activities in relation to others.

(2) What is the usual pattern of adaptation?

Studies have shown, in a variety of contexts, that the way in which a person adapts to change in later life will reflect the way in which he has been accustomed to adapt in earlier life. One of the major factors found to affect the ability to adjust to relocation in old age, for example, is 'the pattern of the individual's prior mastery' (Yawney and Slover 1973). People who have coped well in the past can usually cope well in future stress situations if they can appraise the situation realistically. If this is a generally applicable assumption, and it does not seem unreasonable to believe that it is, then assessment of the individual should include some measure (estimation and evaluation) of his adaptive patterns. Such measures do not seem to be available with a high degree of reliability, although it may be possible in a research context to predict adaptation to some specific situations (Bloom and Blenkner 1970). Such an assessment is generally reliant on theoretical assumptions and subjective interpretations but can be informed by experience and practice wisdom. One method which does begin to develop an understanding of the individual's approach to life has been called the life review (Butler 1963). Although primarily developed as a way of using the individual's reminiscences in a process of therapy, life history taking has been increasingly used in the research context. It may prove equally useful in the service delivery context: an understanding of the adaptive capacities of older people and their usual problem-solving approaches can be developed through discussion of their past life and significant events in it.

(3) How dependent are they?

This may be seen in two ways. First, people may be objectively dependent on others for help with physical needs or because of deterioration in intellectual ability. Second, most people are involved in relationships and interactions with others which are subjectively defined: dependence relates as much to what people are prepared to do and are allowed to do as to objective measures of capacity. Considerable efforts have been made to develop appropriate measures of dependence (see e.g. Pattie and Gilleard 1979; Schiphorst 1979; Booth 1980) and to begin to relate assessment of the needs of the older person to assumptions and expectations about the general usage of resources. They are concerned, in other words, with the match between needs and provisions as well as with assessing the individual.

(4) What is the relationship between abilities and the environment?

Another way of expressing this question is to ask whether people are in the right place. Some detailed work on the environment and the individual has been developed (Lawton 1980). Many older people are in institutions not because their abilities are less than those of many others in the community but because the environment − both physical (poor housing, low income, frailty and ill-health) and social (lack of family, friends, and neighbours) − in which they were living created too great a stress for them to continue to cope. An obvious conclusion must be that more appropriate environments would prevent admission. It also follows that if older people are to leave care the environment to which they move must be carefully constructed to match individual abilities and provisions and resources and to reduce the environmental pressure.

(5) What are the risks of change?

It has been very well established that moving from one place to another is at best stressful and potentially damaging for older people (Brearley *et al.* 1980). Researchers have considered movement between various forms of accommodation and found that the potential for negative consequences seems to exist independently of the kind of accommodation. Tobin and Lieberman (1976), although writing about the American context, noted that those who stay in nursing homes for a short period are especially vulnerable. This has important implications for the present discussion: we do not know enough about which people are most vulnerable to such changes, but those who are physically and mentally frail, and those who feel that change is forced on them, are very likely to be at risk during movement.

One factor which does seem to be relevant is the quality of the environment to which people are moving. The danger to an old lady who stays in a convalescent home for a few weeks following hospital treatment before returning home to live alone in a cold, damp house will be much greater than that to someone discharged from residential care to sheltered housing with a high level of formal support services and a network of family and friends.

(6) Who makes the decisions?

It was established in the earlier section of this book that we believe that positive planning for the use of residential care begins before admission. This does not mean that the decision is made solely by the field-worker with the older person and his family. If it is true, as has been argued here, that positive planning involves matching needs and environment then it follows that those with the best knowledge of resources should be involved in assessment and decision-making. The residential worker should therefore be involved with the older person as early as possible in planning and decision-making. Although this has been advocated for some time there is little substantial evidence that it does happen consistently. Impressionistically, however, there seems to be an increased acceptance of the importance of shared decision-making (older person − family − field-worker − residential worker) and some Social Services

Departments have developed the principle in practice. Most, for instance, have accepted that wherever possible the older person should visit the home before a final decision and some expect the residential worker to visit him in his own home, and some have begun to establish short-term assessment homes to ensure that full investigation is carried out (see e.g. Roberts 1981).

The preliminary decision and plan should therefore develop around thorough assessment, which involves the older person and those who provide care for him as well as field-workers and residential workers. When people are living in the institutional situation it is sometimes easy for initiative to be surrendered in the increased dependence on others and it is therefore particularly important to provide continuing review and reassessment which encourages and enables the older person to retain control of decisions about his own life.

REVIEW AND REHABILITATION

So far this discussion has been generally concerned with older people needing residential care in a longer-term perspective. Two other groups are important: those admitted for short stays in old people's homes and those admitted for hospital treatment. In such cases it seems just as important to have a planned and purposeful approach, since there is an opportunity for a detailed consideration of the most appropriate form of care. Of course the fact that an old lady is admitted to a home for two weeks while her daughter takes a holiday is no justification for intrusive medical screening or detailed mental testing: which of us wants to be asked to repeat the alphabet backwards and name the Prime Minister during our annual holiday! Nevertheless for many people a systematic approach to discussing their needs and way of life can help in planning an improved environment on their return home.

It would not be appropriate to give detailed consideration here to rehabilitation approaches in residential care and elsewhere and excellent reviews already exist (see e.g. Leeming 1979; Davies and Knapp 1981). There is substantial agreement that good rehabilitation is based on a multidisciplinary approach and the importance of teamwork has been stressed by most authorities in both planning and rehabilitation. Although there is some reason to question whether team discussions are as effective as their advocates claim (Fairhurst 1977; Rowlings 1978) the ideal of shared decision-making continues to be an attractive principle for practice.

In considering rehabilitation some further questions become relevant:

(1) How can people be helped to improve?

The earlier discussion of assessment has shown that improvement cannot be a matter only of better health, or curing illness, but must also be related to the individual's ability to perform specific tasks. This in turn must be related to the environment and the question of whether he can do what is necessary to survive in his present environment – or in the proposed environment.

(2) How can people be helped to learn or relearn skills?

This question therefore becomes of central importance. To take a simple (and necessarily over-simplified) example: if an old man has deteriorated in health and has had to be admitted to hospital because of his inability to cook a hot meal, it may be a relatively easy matter to provide him with a list of nutritious food (and someone to buy it for him) and to help him relearn the basic skills of kettle and cooker. He can then return home to the same physical environment but with improved skills to manage that environment.

The answer to these questions about improvement and learning are vital but it is not appropriate to deal with them here. The reader is recommended to consult some of the recent excellent texts in the field: Sections 5 and 6 of the Open University reader edited by Carver and Liddiard (1978) and the associated units of the Open University course 'An Ageing Population'; the social work books by Lowy (1979) and by Rowlings (1981) and the more specialized book on social work and mental infirmity by Gray and Isaacs (1979) will all be helpful.

(3) Where can people go?

There seems little point discussing rehabilitation without relating this to specific outcome goals which will be expressed partly in terms of future environments. Some of the most important issues have been set out in the early part of this chapter. Although choice is important as a principle for practice with older people, in reality it is often severely restricted because of the inflexibility and inadequacies of the formal resources that are available. A number of innovations have been developed but few of these have been extended sufficiently widely to be generally recommended. One of the most widely reported, and certainly the most thoroughly monitored, is the scheme developed in Kent to provide a package of care for people living in the community which will give a level of support sufficient to prevent admission to care (Challis and Davies, 1980). By careful interweaving of formal and informal services by social workers acting as case planners and co-ordinators, it has been possible to maintain older people at home, and this seems to point the way towards the only realistic view of older people leaving care. Only if it is possible to create an extensive and intensive set of supports in the community will it be possible for older people to return. This will inevitably involve a considerable amount of planning and effort for the worker involved − whether it be the residential worker or the field-worker. It also depends entirely on the availability of alternative accommodation.

The kinds of accommodation which are likely to be available to older people who have given up their own homes are obviously very limited. For some the prospect of moving to live with family may be one possibility and that may provide the physically safest course of action, although not necessarily the most successful. Sheltered housing or perhaps the use of peripatetic wardens to provide support for the more isolated would also seem logical alternatives for those who do not require the levels of care provided in residential care, but there is little evidence of anything but very occasional moves of this nature. A further prospect may be placement in private households. For many years some local authorities and voluntary agencies have attempted to develop assisted lodgings schemes but it has only been relatively recently that these have been given substantial support or monitoring. A survey of such schemes, conducted nationally, found that about a third of long-term placements in assisted lodgings arise from relocation of elderly people from institutions. These relocations were not only from old people's homes but also from psychiatric and subnormality hospitals and tended to involve people inappropriately placed in the first instance (Thornton and Moore 1980). Although relatively small numbers of people are involved in such placements recent limited success suggests that it may be possible to extend this approach for some people.

Those older people who expect to be in hospital or old people's homes for only a short period will normally be returning to their previous, familiar environment, but a number of issues may also arise here. If they live alone the house may be cold, damp, and unwelcoming, and it may require adaptation to meet changed needs, as, for example, after a stroke illness. If the older person is returning to live with family it may be that the space − physical or emotional − which he occupied has begun to close: the bedroom converted back into a lounge, the commode put away in the garage, or perhaps more seriously the grandchildren have discovered the relief of having more space, freedom to make a lot of noise, etc. There may be a need for help from social workers in many different ways to help with the preparation of both the older person and the place and people to which he will return. In fact one survey of social workers found the aspect of their work which created the most difficult problems in arranging hospital discharge was in dealing with relatives (Age Concern Greater London 1980).

A more detailed discussion of accommodation options for older people wishing to be housed near relatives is available and is recommended (Tinker 1980). Tinker outlines five accommodation options: small units (usually a flat or bungalow); housing divided up into flats; sheltered housing; others such as

Granny Annexes, prefabricated or mobile homes; and extra support in their own home. In concluding her discussion of options she makes several important recommendations, including providing more advice and information; providing more small accommodation; considering ways of sheltering older people in their own houses (alarm systems, peripatetic wardens, good neighbouring, etc.); granting transfer of tenancies for those wishing to move nearer relatives and making dwellings more readily available for older people from outside housing catchment areas; not debarring owner-occupiers from council accommodation; using and developing housing association provision; considering exchange systems; and making decisions more open. If some of these options become more freely available it will be more realistically possible to plan for leaving residential accommodation.

CONTINUITY AND AFTER-CARE

Continuity can be maintained in many ways. Initial planning and review with a key worker will provide a through link which must be maintained. Some people may be able to move to live in a flat with support from community services and day care or intermittent care in the residential home in which they previously stayed.

The most substantial work on after-care arrangements and the elderly has been produced in relation to hospital discharge, which is hardly surprising since many more people leave hospital than leave homes. The same general principles seem relevant to both settings. A report of the Continuing Care Project (Slack and Gibbins 1979), which was established to improve the quality of support and care in the community for elderly people discharged from hospital, makes a number of very important recommendations. The report stresses the need for a planned policy for all discharges which ensures that plans for leaving begin early in the patient's hospital stay. Regular interdisciplinary meetings and the sharing of information are also advocated along with regular monitoring of arrangements and the need for good communication with patient and relatives (Slack and Gibbins 1979).

Once again, it is not necessary to discuss principles of good practice in after-care in detail here: the literature already quoted gives a thorough introduction to social work in the community. The point to be emphasized here is the need to maintain a link between the residential and the community experience. To place an older person in residential care for a few weeks of 'rest and recuperation' may have some short-term benefits but these must be consolidated in a continuing plan. Equally, no older person should be left to survive without support after a long period in care: the readjustment to independent living is likely to require considerable help which may involve both field and residential workers.

SUMMARY

This review has, of necessity, been generalized and rather abstract because it is concerned with what should and could be done for older people leaving residential care rather than what social workers actually do – other than in relatively few, isolated and exceptional cases. Often this is realistic: it has been shown here that most older people in residential care are very old and frail and have probably arrived there in stressful circumstances with no expectation of ever moving again.

But there is reason to believe that some people in old people's homes do have sufficient skills and abilities to be able to cope in a less protected and less restrictive environment. For some of these change is not possible because they do not wish to move and would be made anxious and distressed by any suggestion that they should. For others, however, it may be that they do not move because they are not aware of the possibilities and current practices do not make them aware. In the end it is probably more realistic to think in terms of putting more people into residential care with an expectation that they may improve and be able to move on. To do this appropriately demands a high level of skill and detailed assessment at the time of admission.

Those older people who enter residential care or hospital for a short stay should also be involved in systematic and careful planning for their discharge as early as possible.

For all those who do wish to move on from institutional living to a more independent existence it does seem from recent research evidence and practical social work knowledge that this will often be most appropriately managed through a package of interwoven services. The breakdown of older people and consequent need for residential care often occurs as a result of the collapse of the main supporting person. The safest support system is therefore likely to be one which does not rest on only one caring agent — or if it does then that carer should receive sufficient support from services to reduce the likelihood of unexpected collapse.

As was suggested in the early part of the book, three factors are of central importance:

(1) Planning and assessment from as early in the process of admission to institutional care as possible.
(2) Continuing review and involvement of the older person in decision-making.
(3) The careful construction of a detailed plan for leaving and for after-care which maintains a sense and reality of continuity in the life of the older person.

Finally, it must be remembered that the great majority of people do not return home: most older people who enter long-term care will die in the institutional setting. That this chapter has not dealt in detail with the part played by death, and anticipation and preparation for death is not to underplay its enormous importance in the residential setting. Residential workers have a considerable part to play in helping older people to plan for departure through death. This should be borne in mind even though it has not been seen as central to the argument presented in this chapter.

6 Mental Hospitals
Jim Black

INTRODUCTION

Mental hospitals are institutional systems of care and treatment. However, the degree to which they are concerned in the processes of integration and repair, holding and maintenance, integrity and growth, and the extent to which these sometimes conflicting goals are pursued and balanced, needs to be understood within this specific context. In this respect, mental hospitals are required to fulfil a number of functions on a continuum from secure custodial care to active therapy in the treatment and control of people with mental health problems. The legal framework, outlining the civil liberties of patients admitted to hospital under compulsory orders, has been described in Chapter 2 and will not be restated here. While these patients represent a significant and important minority, the majority of patients in hospital are not there against their will. Hence, this chapter takes a broader view within which the termination of a compulsory order would be one necessary element to be considered for facilitating discharge from hospital for those individuals involved.

In describing social work within this institution and the social worker's contribution to the process of discharge, it is necessary to remember that social work, in this setting, is complicated by factors beyond the relationship between an individual patient's needs and the ability of a social worker situated within the hospital to meet them. Thus, the achievement of positive planning leads us to consider elements beyond the practice of social work. Hence, we will be concerned with both planning at the national and local level and, within the institution, interdisciplinary co-operation and work. Not only are social workers working in mental hospitals employed by an agency external to their place of work, but also their ability to control the care and treatment process is subject to factors unique to this environment. Thus, this chapter starts by identifying some of the constraints on role performance from factors external to day-to-day practice. It then proceeds to consider the negotiation of the social work role within the medical team and within this context identifies a social worker's contribution in the process of discharge planning and after-care in respect of two case examples.

SOCIAL POLICY AND POSITIVE PLANNING

An understanding of the importance of the boundaries set by social policy as it affects positive discharge planning is best illustrated by a brief historical account of the development of two related themes which have underpinned the planning of mental health services in Great Britain in the last quarter-century: 'community care' and 'service integration'.

The deinstitutionalization of the mentally ill and the development of community-based services, encompassing district-based psychiatric health services and a range of residential and day care facilities provided by local authorities was first outlined in the Report of the Royal Commission in 1957 (HMSO 1957). This goal, to replace the Victorian mental hospitals and to promote a shift in emphasis from hospital to community care, remains the central objective of policy and it has been restated with varying levels of enthusiasm in subsequent White Papers and policy statements. The high point of optimism, 1962, saw the publication of the Hospital Plan (MoH 1962) which predicted that the mental hospital population would be halved by 1975 with a transfer of 75,000 patients to community care, the closing of half the psychiatric beds, and the integration of the majority of psychiatric services in to general hospitals. However, by the target date, the White Paper 'Better Services for the Mentally Ill' (DHSS 1975), while accepting that such expectations had not been fulfilled, reiterated the validity of pursuing those objectives. Reviewing the fifteen years since the passing of the 1959 Mental Health Act, the White Paper stated:

> 'We believe that the failures and problems are at the margins and that the basic concept remains valid . . . for the future the main aims must be the development of much more locally based services, and a shift in the balance between hospital and social services care.'
>
> (Para. 2.17, DHSS 1975)

Between the passing of the 1959 Act and the publication of the White Paper 'progress had been made'. More patients were being treated in the community. The length of stay of patients in hospital had been reduced and a substantial number of 'long-stay patients' who had been institutionalized in the past had been discharged. However, commenting on the rehabilitation and resettlement of this group the document points to the slow development of community facilities. Undoubtedly, the slow growth of suitable alternatives − for instance, by 1975 only 43 per cent of the minimum recommended places in hostels were being provided by local authority or private schemes − hampered the effective achievement of policy goals (Royal College of Psychiatrists 1980). However, an allied factor was an increasing critical awareness of the need to monitor and evaluate the outcomes of active discharge policies. Research was, and is, continuing to draw attention to the fact that while a large group of people with severe and disabling mental illnesses live outside hospital, community facilities do not take the most severely handicapped (Hewett, Ryan, and Wing 1975), that families receiving a discharged relative home are given the minimum of support (Creer and Wing 1974) and that a significant number of discharged patients are living in hostels for the destitute or just sleeping rough (Leach and Wing 1978). This has led commentators to question the quality of life and care provided outside the hospital and to raise doubts that discharge *to* the community has effectively integrated those patients involved into community living. Furthermore, other writers have pointed to the emergence of new groups of long-stay patients within the hospital population (Mann and Cree 1976). What had gone wrong?

While the damaging effects of institutional life and the stigmatizing effect of segregation of the mentally ill had underpinned this movement to restructure services radically (and eventually to close the mental hospitals), other policy objectives and financial constraints on public spending have placed limits on the achievement of comprehensive community-based services for the mentally ill. Let us examine these two factors, for without positive planning at the national level the realization of policy objectives in the local context becomes problematic.

Three major administrative reforms of the late sixties and early seventies radically reshaped the organizational framework within which the development of integrated community-based services for the mentally ill were to be achieved: the creation of Social Service Departments in 1971; the reorganization of local authority boundaries in 1974; and in the same year the administrative reorganization of the Health Service. One commentator reflecting on these changes contends that their prime consequence, far from leading towards service integration and coordination, was to destroy the unity of the mental health services (Jones 1979).

'The extraordinary thing is that it had all been done in the name of "integration". Psychiatric social work had been integrated into generic social work. Psychiatrists had been integrated into general medicine. Psychiatric hospitals had been integrated into the general hospital system. The only people who remained unintegrated were the mentally ill, who were now required to carve their needs into neat parcels labelled 'medical' and 'social' and to apply to the appropriate authority for care and treatment.'

(Jones 1979:10)

While it is not intended to debate the reasons underlying these major changes here, it is certain that they had the effect of destroying or changing many of the long-standing and developing relationships between various people working in the mental health field. However, of equal importance was the effect of these organizational changes taken together with the financial constraints placed on government spending over the last decade. In this respect, the elements of the mental health services existing in health and local authorities have had to compete with other pressing demands from other medical specialisms or client groups. For both authorities faced with under-financing, the development of services for the mentally ill has become a relatively minor interest.

MIND in its evidence to the Royal Commission on the National Health Service sees the need for government to recognize and redress this position if the policy objectives set out in the 1975 White Paper are to be realized (MIND 1977). While Joint Funding, the only device which emerged in the late seventies to divert expenditure towards community care, primed the faltering attempts at Joint Care Planning between health and local authorities into a more effective machinery, the achievement of integrated district-based services and the development of the principle of 'community care' are formidable. Under-financing of both sectors, coupled with the upheavals of administrative reform, has not promoted positive planning either at the national or area level. The fact that progress has been made points to the commitment of individual professionals and managers at the local level to overcome these problems.

Present policy initiatives seem still to be striving for a formula to provide a co-ordinating framework for planning between health and social services. The consultative document, 'Care in the Community' (DHSS 1981b), which discusses some ingenious ways of removing some of the barriers to transferring patients from in-patient health care to social service community care, suggests that in a time of financial retrenchment new policy initiatives are necessary if any progress can be made. Furthermore, the idea contained in the document, that a single agency might take prime responsibility for a particular group of patients, seems to be an admission that the existing planning framework in which health and local authorities operate has not effected the desired shift in resources towards community care.

This necessarily brief overview of the social policy framework with regard to two major themes in the development of mental health services is illustrative of the difficulties of achieving positive planning at the national and, in consequence, at the local level. It has also laid the policy context within which the discharge of mental patients is set. It is evident that while policy objectives espouse the principles of 'community care' and the development of integrated services, other objectives and financial constraints have placed considerable barriers on their achievement. The social worker operating within the mental hospital is not only constrained through the limited nature or lack of community provision in effectively planning the departure of certain patients but also, being an employee of the local authority, is in the position of being at the interface between the two agencies in day-to-day work.

THE INSTITUTIONAL AND ORGANIZATIONAL SETTING

How far does the very nature of the mental hospital prepare patients for return to community life? Two different theoretical perspectives provide us with an understanding of both the institutional experience for a person within, or passing through, the care and treatment system and the organizational context of social work practice in this setting.

In his classic study of the mental hospital as a total institution Goffman presents a view of a closed system in which the acceptance of the patient role and the processes of care and treatment have the effect of reducing an individual's capability for managing the everyday world outside when he is discharged (Goffman 1961). At the point of admission a person not only enters an institutional world which is different from and closed to the society from which he has been removed, but also the process of admission confronts him with a status passage through which he acquires the status of 'mental patient' (Scheff 1966). Elements of the ethos of the institution to which he now belongs include: acceptance of a passive and sick role, acceptance of the power of medical and nursing staff to control his activity, and limitations on his ability to manage his personal as opposed to his patient identity. Everyday activities occur within a single location and communal living is the norm within the environment of the ward. Day-to-day routines are at variance with the world outside and this distinctive milieu develops its own closed culture.

For Goffman, the longer a person is exposed to this ethos the more likely it is that he will accept the reality of life in hospital and absorb the values and roles associated with it. The end result is 'disculturation', the loss of the capacity to manage, albeit temporarily, the social world outside the institution. On leaving the hospital, this process of cultural adaptation operates in reverse. But it is more complex, necessitating a move from a relatively protective and circumscribed social environment to a world in which the mental patient role has a stigmatizing effect and in which role expectations are more problematic and subject to negotiation.

While Goffman's interpretation has been criticized from various quarters (Smith 1970; Siegler and Osmond 1971), the 'institutional effects' of the social environment of the hospital and the patient role are generally recognized as placing constraints on the successful return of patients to the community. Building on his work in this country, other writers have described the significant relationship between the institutional ethos and the limits it places on the capacity of the institution to rehabilitate and resettle patients (see e.g. Brown *et al.* 1966; King, Raynes, and Tizard 1971; Jones 1974). Certainly these disabling effects, stemming from the treatment and caring process, operate to a greater or lesser extent for all patients within or passing through the system.

Does this perspective, with its emphasis on the institution as a closed system, represent the typical features of British mental hospitals today? It could be argued that the unintended consequences of institutional care and treatment have been recognized and with the emphasis on 'open door' policies, community-based services, informal admission, and shorter lengths of stay, the banner goals of mental hospitals are essentially therapeutic rather than custodial in nature. A second theoretical perspective adds to our understanding of these conflicting functions of hospital care and treatment. Furthermore, it points to features of the organizational context which set their own boundaries on social work within the hospital. For Vinter, mental hospitals are one example of treatment organizations and have as their primary function the alteration of the behaviour and/or personality of their clientele (Vinter 1963). While the aim of changing people is dominant, the hospital being a complex organization has a hierarchy of goals. Thus, while having a primary commitment to therapeutic treatment, mental hospitals may also serve as both residential and, to a lesser extent, custodial systems of care for a certain clientele.

Treatment organizations are concerned with solving problems of deviance. Thus, from this perspective, mental hospitals serve patients who have demonstrated that they have 'defective attributes' or are 'improperly motivated' and hence are not able adequately to perform conventional social roles. While in the past the response to such behaviour was to exclude or remove the person to custodial care, today there is an expectation and optimism that deviance, and specifically deviance characterized as mental illness, can be treated. Thus the potential for the successful rehabilitation of the mentally ill is generally accepted as the mental hospitals' primary goal and this underpins the treatment philosophies employed by change agents operating within them. Central to Vinter's perspective is that treatment organizations employ various occupational groups who claim to possess the technical competences necessary to this primary goal. His thesis is that treatment organizations can be differentiated on technical dimensions. However, this need not concern us here. What is important is that this analysis enables us to understand some of the complexities within role relationships which stem from the shared, but sometimes conflicting, treatment philosophies of those occupational groups employed by the hospital to treat and rehabilitate patients.

Mental hospitals rely on a number of occupational groups who have developed expertise and skill which can be employed in the treatment of their clientele. Psychiatrists, nurses, psychologists, occupational therapists, and social workers typically operate within this setting. Each group has developed expertise in relation to mental health problems but it is the first two who both espouse and maintain the dominant treatment philosophy employed. This philosophy, 'the medical model', is centred round diagnosis, treatment, and prognosis of illness. Diagnosis, the identification of a specific mental illness or syndrome, determines the nature of the problem, and treatment consists of drug, physical, milieu or psychotherapy under the direction of a psychiatrist accompanied by nursing care. Prognosis in this area of medicine is attempted, but accepted as problematic. However, there is an assumption that medical science will advance and such judgements will be made with more certainty in the future. This model, in its ideal type, would define the skills of psychologists, occupational therapists, and social workers as 'auxiliary' or 'para-medical' and thus to be employed by the doctor as a constituent part of medical intervention. To a greater or lesser extent, individual practitioners within these other disciplines accept the assumptions upon which the medical model is founded. However, no one working within the care and treatment system can operate without acknowledging the dominance of medical intervention and the superior power position vested in the doctor role. This position is not only legitimated by the legal and social policy framework but also reflects the beliefs and expectations of both patients and the majority of people outside the institution. Furthermore,the bureaucratic organization of the hospital explicitly acknowledges the primacy of medical personnel. Work is separated into professional, i.e. medical, and administrative spheres. In the former, control over the regulation of treatment and medical competence is vested in medical peers within the institution – consultants, who are in a powerful strategic position *vis-à-vis* patients, colleagues and other occupational groups (Smith 1958; Goss 1963).

The degree to which other treatment philosophies survive and prosper within the hospital seems to be dependent on two factors – first, how far they can be accommodated to this dominant medical orientation and second, whether they receive patronage from medical personnel (Goldie 1977). Through these mechanisms diverse philosophies such as, for example, behavioural and analytic psychology have co-existed with the medical model in hospitals. Furthermore, orientations based on psychological models have been used, through patronage, to experiment with radical changes to ward regimes – for example, token economy programmes (see Ayllon and Azrin 1968; Liberman 1971) and milieu therapy (Jones 1968). Some of the attempts to accommodate these different treatment philosophies in the rehabilitation of schizophrenic patients have led two commentators to suggest that some programmes use models which, at the theoretical level, lack any comprehensible relation to each other, and 'which if seriously and consistently applied would have diverse and mutually incompatible consequences' (Siegler and Osmond 1966:1193). A further complicating factor is that these 'minor' philosophies cannot be differentiated on the basis of a particular discipline. For example behavioural psychology, the principles of which are employed primarily by clinical psychologists, is also the basis upon which social workers (Hudson 1978) and nurses (Marx *et al.* 1975) have operated.

From the limited empirical evidence available, social workers in mental hospitals seem typically to accept the medical model as the prime treatment philosophy (Goldie 1977; Stevenson and Parsloe 1978). This not only places doctors and nurses in a key position in the treatment of individual patients but also tends to give them the discretion in identifying those patients who would benefit from social work intervention. Furthermore, medical rather than social work judgements set the priorities and focus of work. In this respect, the common practice of attaching individual social workers to a medical team clearly limits social work's ability to set its own priorities within the institution.

To quote from Stevenson and Parsloe:

'This was most clearly illustrated in the English Psychiatric Hospital: there was little medical treatment in some chronic wards and so social work involvement was also limited. Yet, it could be argued that the need presented by such wards might call for more social work rather than medical involvement.'

(Stevenson and Parsloe 1978:281)

This is not to suggest that tensions do not exist in this position. Obviously, the fact that social workers are employed by an outside agency raises the question of their relationship to the Health Service in general and more particuarly their accountability to the medical team. However, freedom to act independently, that is, without the prior sanction of medical and nursing personnel, is limited and the dominance of medical treatment in British mental hospitals cannot be denied.

ROLE NEGOTIATION WITHIN THE MEDICAL TEAM

We have seen that certain boundaries are placed round social work in mental hospitals which are produced by factors external to the transactions of a social worker and his client. Social policy, the unintended consequences of institutional care and treatment, and the organizational constraints set by the dominance of medical treatment, all in differing ways circumscribe social work's ability to set its own priorities in this institutional setting. However, while *social work's* objective control over institutional processes is limited, the *individual social worker's* contribution towards treatment and discharge planning is more complex. For while psychiatrists lay claim to a general mandate to manage treatment and care, their position is one of incorporating rather than excluding other disciplines in decision-making (Goldie 1977). Hence, an individual social worker's freedom to participate in both planning and treatment necessarily needs to be understood within the context of the medical team.

'The multi-professional team', 'interdisciplinary working', and 'the specialist therapeutic team' have been terms employed to describe team-work in which two or more disciplines come together to co-ordinate and work in concert to some prescribed goal (DHSS 1975; BASW 1979; Royal College of Psychiatrists 1980). For instance, in exhorting team-work the 1975 White Paper sees team-working as of 'utmost importance' and 'that staff should recognise the potential value of multi-professional working and be ready to adopt this approach whenever it is in the patient's best interests' (DHSS 1975:21). Today, team membership is the norm for the majority of mental hospital social workers. They are typically attached to a consultant, a group of wards or a specialist unit and this usually involves one worker undertaking all 'the social work' coming from this work setting. Dependent on the locus of work, its range is potentially very wide but as Goldie reports, the activities taken on by individual workers are subject to negotiation (Goldie 1977). In this respect, this writer points to the differing ideological positions of team members, rather than their treatment philosophies, as being critical to their sense of freedom in decision-making and their constructed role. Workers who see themselves as auxiliaries to psychiatrists define their role differently from those who strive towards a complementary relationship or those who take a dissident stance. Hence, the role negotiated by the individual worker is vital if social work is to contribute to treatment and discharge planning.

From this position, it is necessary to consider whether, as some writers have argued, team-working is primarily concerned with negotiating status relationships and asserting occupational claims to certain activities rather than a way of co-ordinating and concerting action towards the well-being or treatment of patients. For Dingwell (Dingwell 1980), to take one critic as an example, team-work 'ultimately fails' since the power and generalized expertise claimed by medicine prevents other disciplines from competing on equal terms to areas of work within their competence encompassed by this broad remit.

To quote Dingwell:

'For the doctors, with their strong sense of individual responsibility, the metaphor is in Webb's terms, that of a football team where they are captain, manager and coach. For the others, with their sense of special expertise, the metaphor is that of the tennis team, a democratic or collegiate group of complementary experts.'

(Dingwell 1980:133)

This analysis leads us to consider two questions. Does team-work provide a better standard of care and treatment for patients? And second, without some redress of the unequal status and power positions of team members, is participative decision-making possible? To some extent the answer to the first question is found in the second where care and treatment planning is negotiated. As Bucher and Stelling (1969) point out, role negotiation is a continuous process and a negotiated consensus is usually arrived at by team members for each case. However, this is only a partial answer, if the objective is to maximize team effectiveness towards an individual patient's needs. As others have argued (Rowbottom and Hey 1978; Webb and Hobdell 1980), planning should be goal-directed towards this end. Thus, as in other care and treatment settings, client participation, either directly or indirectly, in team members' acknowledgement of the patients' definitions of their needs should, wherever possible, lead team members' interventions. Equally, in the substantial grey areas where no one discipline has either the self-evident expertise or resources from its occupational mandate, a decision has to be arrived at by the team that the doctor *or* the social worker *or* the nurse *or* the psychologist might have the individual qualities, skills, or experience to serve a particular patient. Thus, with these prescriptions, occupational rivalry could be channelled constructively in team decision-making. This essentially pragmatic approach seems to be the basis upon which effective team-working can operate so long as the psychiatrist involved fulfils an accommodating role.

THE SOCIAL WORK ROLE IN DISCHARGE PLANNING AND AFTER-CARE

Significantly, a central thrust of team-work in mental hospitals is geared towards the discharge of patients. However, the meaning of leaving the hospital can be very different for the individuals concerned. For some, it may mean a return to a familiar environment from which they were recently admitted; while for others, it might involve a move to a new residential setting in which their care and/or treatment will continue to be under the supervision of hospital or social services staff. The following discussion examines the elements of planning and after-care with reference to two case examples drawn to illustrate team working and the activities undertaken by a social worker in respect of these two outcomes. The process rather than the methods employed will be our major concern.

It is our conviction that discharge planning is a vital component for consideration for all patients leaving the hospital. Hence, the constituent parts of this process – positive planning, review, preparation, departure, and after-care are equally applicable to other situations.

The case of Mrs Jones

Our first example illustrates the case of a patient who can be seen to have a relatively short attachment to the hospital's treatment and care system. The setting is an acute admission ward in a typical mental hospital. The treatment team includes a consultant psychiatrist with a positive orientation towards other disciplines, the nursing staff of the ward, and a social worker who views himself in a complementary role *vis-à-vis* other disciplines. Other occupational groups, for example clinical psychologists and community nurses, are called upon if required. The team meets together weekly to assess and plan treatment and to decide on whether a patient can leave the hospital.

Mrs Jones was admitted informally from the casualty ward of the general hospital. It is her first experience in mental hospital. She attempted suicide by taking a mixture of tablets prescribed by her general practitioner for depression and anxiety. The sister in charge of the ward becomes aware that the patient is worried about her children and is not settling on the ward. She refers the case to the social worker to investigate and assess the home environment prior to the meeting.

The social worker's first step on receipt of the referral is to interview the patient. This serves a number of functions. It initiates a data collection process which will contribute to multidisciplinary decision-making. It will investigate the immediate problem identified by the nursing staff and it will be the beginning of the social worker's own intervention in the case. As

Mrs Jones has not previously come face to face with a social worker before, it will be necessary for him to explain his role and position in the hospital and within the treatment team. In this respect his explanation is set on a general level with a view to gaining her co-operation. Whether an initial contract is formed between the social worker and Mrs Jones is dependent on his interviewing skills. His initial focus is directed on her immediate concern − her children.

The social worker is already aware from the medical file of the account of the events leading to admission, Mrs Jones's life and medical history and the preliminary diagnosis which led to the decision to admit her. He has also inquired whether she or her children are known to area team colleagues. They are not. However, he knows that by listening and sharing with her an account of her immediate crisis the foundations could be laid to the formation of a relationship for future work. From this interview the social worker will begin to make sense of Mrs Jones's predicament and to make an initial assessment which he can use as a basis for preliminary action. He finds that his client wishes to discharge herself; she says she feels better, is worried about how her husband is looking after her children, and wants to return to her family. It is clear that Mrs Jones's major concern is to return home. However, without more information and consultation with other team members he is not prepared to consider this option seriously. He thus decides to take a holding strategy and explains that first she would need to see the doctor. He knows that patients generally 'seek permission' before discharging themselves, and that he neither has the mandate to take the decision on his own nor is he convinced that he could advocate to this end on behalf of his client without knowing the hazards and dangers for her at home. The risks involved cannot be assessed. At this point Mrs Jones breaks down and in the remaining part of the interview gives her account of her problems.

Thus the social worker starts to build up a picture of the events precipitating Mrs Jones's attempted suicide, her familial and social circumstances, and her immediate problems. By the end of the interview his initial assessment points strongly to marital and financial problems. Mrs Jones's worries concerning her children seem to be based on her anxiety that her husband might not be looking after them adequately. This, coupled with her fears that she will be treated with electro-convulsive therapy, seem to be her immediate reasons for her wish to return home. With her agreement, the social worker decides to make a home visit to reassure her and himself that the children are being looked after and to complete his initial social work assessment. He is also able to tell her that the consultant psychiatrist in charge of her medical treatment rarely uses ECT to treat depression and that she has the right to refuse treatment if she wishes. He reports the outcome of his interview to the ward sister.

By the time the ward team meeting takes place, the social worker has made his home visit, identified that the children are now being cared for temporarily by the patient's sister, and interviewed Mrs Jones's husband. He has had a second interview with Mrs Jones, and gathered enough data together to make his initial assessment.

The treatment team discuss the case. The psychiatrist is primarily concerned with making a firm diagnosis of the patient's illness and formulating an immediate treatment plan. The social worker, on the other hand, is aware of a marital crisis and financial problems which led to Mrs Jones's attempted suicide, and a number of life events which could have contributed to her actions. He is also aware that the potential to change or ameliorate this situation will be his continuing focus of work with Mrs Jones to prepare and plan her return home. The outcome of joint discussion is a treatment plan based on a two-dimensional approach: drug therapy to treat 'acute reactive depression' and planned social work intervention. However, both the nursing sister and the social worker report that Mrs Jones is adamant that she wants to leave the hospital. None of the team feels that this would be the right decision. The doctor considers that there has been little evidence of an improvement in her mental state, the nurse points to the fact that she is still not settling down on the ward and the social worker would like to start his work within the hospital by building up his relationship with Mrs Jones and holding a joint interview with her and her husband. While the unacceptable risks identified in discharge are jointly held, it is the doctor who is legally responsible for the patient and he takes the ultimate responsibility. He decides to counsel Mrs Jones and explain to her that he will seek a compulsory order if he is unable to convince her that she should remain in hospital.

Compulsory powers are not needed, and Mrs Jones remains an informal but rather unwilling patient for the next six weeks. Further reviews reveal a marked improvement in her mental state. While the psychiatrist considers that drug therapy has been the major factor which has led to this improvement, the social worker has been able to work towards dealing with some of the problems which had led to admission. His joint meetings in the hospital between Mr and Mrs Jones have led to their acceptance that they should work on their marital difficulties and he has been able to provide them with practical advice to help them begin to sort out their financial problems. Mr Jones's luck in finding a new job (he had been unemployed following redundancy) seemed to have been a turning point in the case.

The decision to discharge Mrs Jones was taken under some pressures external to the case because of a waiting list of urgent admissions. The team members agree that her departure should be planned and the social worker is designated prime responsibility for after-care. Mrs Jones leaves the hospital following a short joint interview with the consultant and the social worker. The consultant informs Mrs Jones's general practitioner of her position and will automatically review the case at a follow-up appointment at the outpatient clinic.

In post-discharge interviews the social worker sees himself as offering in the short term a supportive relationship for Mrs Jones. He monitors her mental state, and helps her and her family adapt to her return home. He sees his prime responsibility as providing continuity of care for his client. He continues to work with Mr and Mrs Jones with their financial and marital problems and eventually convinces them that they should seek help from a marriage guidance counsellor. His reasons for transfer are twofold. First, Mrs Jones is discharged from out-patient care at her follow-up clinic appointment. The social worker has reported that her mood has remained stable and that the acute crisis that had been generated in the marriage had been eased significantly by Mr Jones's new job and the regular income it brought into the family. Second, the worker was aware that Mrs Jones identified him with her rather unhappy stay in hospital. This was an appropriate point to terminate his involvement.

Discussion

This case example illustrates some elements of team decision-making on an acute admission ward. While the work of those involved is focused on treatment and care, discharge is an imminent possibility throughout Mrs Jones's stay.

Her experience demonstrated the difficulties of a person on a first admission to a mental hospital. She was not only faced with the problem of making sense of and accounting for her actions to staff, but was also having to cope with her role as patient on the ward. In this respect, non-compliance with the ward regime is interpreted by ward staff as uncooperative behaviour. These experiences added to her anxiety and, coupled with her feelings of separation from her children, she understandably wanted to return to a familiar environment however unsafe it might have appeared to the team members involved with her.

It is worth considering here whether alternative service provision, if it had been available, would have coped with this 'psychiatric emergency' more appropriately. For instance, if Mrs Jones had been transferred to a psychiatric unit within the general hospital some of her anxieties associated with her view of mental hospitals and her difficulties in accepting the patient role might have been minimized. Second, if our team had been geared to providing a community-based crisis service as envisaged in the 1975 White Paper (DHSS 1975) and which has been provided experimentally in some areas (Meacher 1979) some of the team's uncertainties associated with her discharge might have been managed more effectively by risking her discharge home following initial assessment with intensive support. As we have seen earlier in this chapter the development of such services has been hampered by both under-financing and the problems of co-ordinated planning.

This example draws attention to some of the organizational factors which impinge on the social worker's role. First, neither the patient nor the social worker was directly accessible to each other. The nursing staff initiated involvement. However, rather than the social worker accepting the referral at face value, he sought the active participation of Mrs Jones, and focused on her needs rather than the team's need for information to diagnose her illness as his initial goal. By taking this stance, he hoped to intervene by building a consistent relationship with her which was oriented to helping her overcome problems beyond her clinical condition.

His deference to the psychiatrist as a means of holding the patient in hospital and similarly in the ward meeting illustrated both the objective reality of his unequal status position in the decision-making process and the inevitable boundaries he had to accept by virtue of team membership. However, his legitimate role to advocate on the patient's behalf if he had felt her request to leave hospital had been justified was negated by the fact that he was unable to formulate a discharge plan based on his assessment and knowledge of the case at that time.

The process of decision-making described in the team meeting leads us to consider the contribution of the social worker. He functioned as a data collector, assessor, and a potential change agent. The social history he presented at the initial meeting was used with medical and nursing information to decide on diagnosis and a treatment plan. His interventions which predated this meeting enabled him to formulate his own assessment. At the team meeting he was able to negotiate his position and offer both his understanding of the case and his potential contribution to treatment. While in this example the treatment plan presented seemed non-problematic, some difficulty could have arisen if the psychiatrist had considered the use of ECT rather than drug therapy. The social worker would have had to inform the team of Mrs Jones's view and advocated on her behalf.

The theme of departure was evident throughout the case but had different meanings for the central actors involved. For Mrs Jones, leaving the hospital was her initial major objective and team members had to use certain devices to hold her in hospital until they had formulated a plan of treatment. However, her transient attachment to the hospital enabled her to maintain her own personal identity. Ironically, if she had remained a passive and co-operative patient and accepted the ward regime it is probable that she would have been discharged earlier. However, her stance focused the attention of the treatment team on her wish to return home and the potential risks involved. In this respect, the doctor was forced to consider his ultimate clinical responsibility and that Mrs Jones was initially an unknown risk. Thus he erred on the side of caution. The social worker was similarly concerned, his client was unknown to him and his area team colleagues. Hence, central to the team's decision to keep the patient in hospital was to plan positively for her departure. The medical staff wished to treat and monitor her mental condition, while the social worker aimed to work with her with a view to counsel and advise her with her problems and build the foundations of his future work outside the hospital. By the time of her departure the team was in a better position to assess the risks to Mrs Jones on her return home. Furthermore, the social worker had made preparation towards her discharge and provided some continuity of care in his follow-up visits. His decision to transfer the case at the termination of team involvement rather than at some more satisfactory conclusion to planned marital therapy could be disputed. The social worker was aware of his own limitations but equally he saw his work within the remit of the medical team. Thus it was at the point the team withdrew that he transferred the case.

The case of John Smith

Our second case example illustrates discharge planning in a specialist facility, a hospital rehabilitation unit which is designed to prepare patients who are considered to be misplaced in hospital for community living. Thus, the unit's primary goal is to habilitate and resettle patients who, for a combination of medical and social reasons, have become permanent residents of the hospital. Its treatment philosophy is based on the assumption that by identifying the constituent parts of an individual patient's social disabilities resulting from mental illness, it is possible to treat or train him so that he will be better able to manage and achieve a social role on his discharge. The ward regime is geared to pursue this objective and provides a social environment and specialist programmes through which patients can learn or relearn self-care, daily living, social and occupational skills. (See Early 1965; Wing and Brown 1970; Olsen 1979; Wing and Olsen 1979; Royal College of Psychiatrists 1980, for examples of rehabilitation and resettlement initiatives in Great Britain.)

The multi-disciplinary team of the unit includes medical staff with a special interest in rehabilitation, nursing staff who have received training in assessment and habilitation techniques, a clinical psychologist, an occupational therapist, and a social worker. The social worker, while attached to the unit, is not centrally involved in the day-to-day work of the ward. However, her role is vital to our patient and the team as she provides a link with the community and its facilities. Other workers — community psychiatric nurses, residential and field social workers, and disablement resettlement officers — form part of an extended team network and are called upon by the unit as required. As with our previous example the objective is to identify the elements of discharge planning and the social worker's contribution to this process rather than the techniques and methods employed.

John Smith has been a permanent hospital resident for the last two years. He suffered an acute psychotic breakdown in his late teens and has had recurrent admissions to hospital. In the past his mental condition has been controlled by medication and he has returned home to the care of his mother with support from a community psychiatric nurse. His last admission was the outcome of a family crisis which resulted in him being admitted primarily for social rather than medical reasons. A number of attempts have been made to place John home but it has been usual for him to return to the ward, either at his family's or his own insistence. It was the recognition that these attempts were unsuccessful that prompted the ward doctor to refer John to the unit. While his psychotic condition is being treated and is controlled, he is considered to have social disabilities and handicaps which prevent the doctor from arranging his discharge. John is a co-operative patient and accepted his transfer to another ward.

The initial assessment process of the unit serves two functions. It assesses a patient's suitability for rehabilitation and it provides, for successful applicants, a base line upon which their progress can be reviewed in further goal planning. Thus, over the next few weeks, John's clinical history is reviewed and the direct effects of his psychosis on his personality and the existence of any active symptoms identified. His behaviour is observed and assessed, his ability to perform self-care and daily living skills identified, and his occupational history and potential assessed and reviewed. While not directly involved in this assessment process, the social worker holds her first interview with John, visits his mother, and in co-operation with the community nurse prepares a detailed social history and assessment of his social and family circumstances.

When this initial data collection process is complete the unit team have sufficient information to make an assessment of John's 'assets' and 'deficits' and taken with the information on his clinical condition and social circumstances it is decided to accept him on the unit. His disabilities are considerable, he tends to be socially withdrawn and rarely initiates anything on his own; his social and daily living skills are limited and his ability to perform simple industrial skills hampered by his lack of concentration. However, the meeting considers his psychosis stable and controlled and that the social work assessment points to John's familiar environment as being unstimulating and often crisis-provoking.

Following this decision, the next stage is for team members to identify both short- and long-term goals which form a basis for John's habilitation. The short-term goals (targets) set are realistic and provide a step-by-step approach to improve John's abilities in self-care, living, social, and work skills, with the long-term objective of raising his level of competence so that it will be possible for him to be discharged from hospital. Targets are reviewed weekly with him and form the basis on which a continual programme of assessment, goal planning, and skill achievement is prepared and monitored by the unit team.

While over the coming months the social worker is not directly involved in the habilitation process, she sees John regularly, with a view to establishing a relationship with him and thus lay a foundation upon which her own role in his discharge will be facilitated. From these interviews and weekly ward meetings she is aware of his progress and is able to contribute her own assessment from her individual counselling. While she and the community nurse have made some attempts to encourage his mother to visit him they are able to confirm the initial pessimistic assessment of his family's ability to support him when he leaves. At this point the unit social worker agrees to take over the responsibility for John's future care as it is probable that he will require a further residential placement on his discharge.

John's progress in the unit is monitored and a point is reached when it is clear that his progress has reached a plateau and it is time to consider his future placement. His assessment points to a marked improvement in his ability to manage his self-care and daily living needs but that his progress in obtaining social skills and in occupational therapy has been slow. Various options are discussed but the available options are severely limited. None are ideally tailored to suit John's personal needs. His willingness to leave is also considered. In this respect the team are aware that the hospital has been his home for nearly three years and the social worker reports that he finds it difficult to consider or comprehend any move away from the now familiar and supportive setting of the unit.

The decision reached is that John's assessment be submitted to the admission panel of the one local authority hostel available in the area which is served by a multi-purpose day centre nearby. The team feels that the hostel will provide him with the supervised setting he needs. Since the unit and hostel staff have developed a controlled introduction process the team hope that John's anxiety and hesitancy to leave the unit might be overcome. The social worker is designated prime responsibility for arranging John's discharge, and she and the ward staff set a target date to prepare John for leaving hospital care.

The application is successful and the social worker works with the ward and residential social work staff to help John to accept this move and to phase his introduction to his new home. The social worker sees her role as co-ordinating his transfer and providing him with a continuous supportive relationship through this period. She arranges introductory meetings for him with the residential social work staff at the hospital, accompanies him on visits to the hostel, and eventually arranges day and overnight stays in the hostel to help him overcome his anxiety and adapt to the idea of moving. His final transfer takes place.

The unit social worker remains John's key worker over the coming weeks until it is evident to her and her residential colleagues that he has begun to settle in. During this period the hostel staff take over his continuing care and designate a residential worker in a 'key role'. The social worker remains in contact with John as part of her liaison role between the unit and the hostel.

Discussion

This second case example describes the work of a unit whose primary aim was to provide a pathway for a patient who had become a permanent resident of the hospital. The unit's very existence is an acknowledgement that the philosophy of treatment and the mental hospital ward regime produces, for certain patients, the negative institutional effects described earlier in this chapter. However, while it provided its own unique social environment within the hospital, the unit nevertheless retained important elements of its institutional setting. Nurses and doctors continued to be the key authority figures for its clientele and the emphasis remained on the pathological features of John's condition — the residual symptoms of his mental illness, its disabling handicaps and the behavioural characteristics of the patient role. However, how far the planned programmes designed to increase his performance and potential addressed the problem of his status passage from 'patient' to 'a member of the community' were questionable. The role models available to him to effect this process of redefinition were severely limited. As others have commented, it is arguable whether a patient's acceptance of his sick role can be tackled within the institution. His significant others remained patients and members of staff. (See Fairweather *et al*. 1969; Lamb *et al*. 1971; Raphael and Peers 1972.) This constraint seems generally to be accepted and current approaches to rehabilitation and resettlement have stressed the need to develop a range of integrated services within and, more particularly, outside the hospital with a view to providing ladders on which patients move to achieve their potential for independent living and meaningful social and economic roles in society (Royal College of Psychiatrists 1980). More realistically, this example was set in a typical local context in which integrated planning has produced few community-based initiatives for the mentally ill.

Within these constraints, how far did the unit and the social worker who was the key to the potential support and caring resources in the community prepare John for his discharge? Certainly the unit's planning was purposeful and goal-directed and worked towards the advancement of John's abilities. Furthermore, short and long-term goals were geared to John's personal needs and the programmes designed were based on a process of continual assessment in which he participated. However, by the time it was decided that he was ready to leave he remained severely disabled in a number of areas. While the unit staff felt that they had reached a plateau, John's readiness to leave was more questionable. The habilitation process, by raising his level of activity and participation in the unit, had produced a strong feeling of attachment to staff and other patients. He was quite naturally hesitant about moving from this micro-environment with its own supporting culture.

This leads us to consider the role of the unit social worker. While she was peripheral to the unit's central activity, she was involved in its decision-making at initial assessment periodic reviews and at formulating the plan of departure. Her role as the gate-keeper for the team to the community was vital to its long-term aims. However, of equal importance was her activity with individual patients. She offered John a supportive relationship while he was in the unit which she maintained until she could partially withdraw at his successful placement. Her actions surrounding the transfer process were presented as an example of the ways in which both hospital and residential staff could co-operate in smoothing a person's pathway to a new residential environment. However, she was faced with two significant problems: John's hesitancy and unwillingness to commit himself to leaving the unit and the limited options that she had available. She considered that, while none of her options was ideal, John's transfer to the hostel was on balance beneficial. The hostel would place him in a situation in which he would need to interact with people who did not take his patient identity for granted. While this placed him under considerable stress initially, this was an acceptable risk which could be controlled by her residential colleagues. Furthermore, she was aware that his new environment would provide him with some degree of protection. Not only would it ascribe to him an intermediate status position between the patient role and the full acceptance of the role as participating member of the community, but also the social milieu of his new setting would provide him with role models which would help him form more normal relationships with other people.

CONCLUSION

The case examples presented illustrate very different experiences for two people who were considered ready to leave a mental hospital. While, in both cases, the opportunity of the social worker to be involved in discharge planning was bounded by the treatment philosophy of the medical team of which he or she was part, it was evident that medical and nursing colleagues were dependent on social work activity and assessment at various stages in the decision-making process. In fact, both Mrs Jones and John Smith required social as well as medical remedies for their problems. It has been shown that a social worker operating within the hospital is placed in a position of having to negotiate his role if he is to intervene effectively with patients. In describing social work within this institution, it has been argued that factors emanating from social policy, the institutional culture and the organizational structure of the hospital affect social work's ability to control the care and treatment process. While traditionally social work with the mentally ill has been focused on work with patients within the community, exhortation of team-working within the institution places them in a situation in which they have to demonstrate both their potential contribution and competence to medical and nursing colleagues who take for granted their dominant role in the treatment and care of patients. In consequence, social workers in this setting require certain specialist skills over and above the relationship which they can offer a patient who becomes their client. These skills include the ability to communicate with other team members; a confidence in their own individual competence and a determination to pursue their own unique contribution to the well-being of patients who become their clients.

7 Conclusion *Paul Brearley*

We have put particular stress throughout this book on the
process of moving through care as the focus for our discussion
of common elements in practice. To concentrate on a process
view is, of course, to recognize the importance of change
through time, and time plays an important part in the experience of institutional living in a number of ways. One of the most
common views of time emphasizes the importance of the individual experience. This view is embodied in many every-day
expressions − 'time hangs heavily', 'time on one's hands', 'a
watched pot never boils', etc. Such a view raises many interesting questions about life in care − how, for instance, does a
young child experience life when his ability to conceive of time
differences is limited and the concept of 'a week' may mean an
eternity or when twenty four hours may feel like a lifetime?
How can a man in hospital cope with carrying on his life when
he can see no clear limit to his stay in the hospital? What do old
people feel about time when they know that they will live in the
same home until a relatively imminent death? Planning for
departure must recognize the importance of the meaning of the
experience of time to the people involved; some may need the
certainty of a fixed departure date while others may only be able
to cope with life in care by operating as if the world outside is
standing still, awaiting their return. It is also important to bear
in mind that an hour each week in the life of a busy social
worker may be experienced very differently from the same hour
in the life of a resident − even though they may spend that time
together.

A contrasting view of time tends to present it as a commodity
to be 'spent', 'given', or allocated in various ways. For most
people time is divided up by routines: work time, leisure time,
meal times, etc. Most may decide for themselves whether to

spend their time on particular activities, or with particular people. In this sense there may not be enough time or there may be too much time – time is 'wasted', 'filled', 'spared', 'killed', etc. Residential living imposes structure on time seen in this perspective; the ways in which time is 'parcelled up' are limited by administrative requirements, for instance, and the freedom of individuals to spend their own time is restricted, just as their freedom to spend their own money is often constrained. Departure may be seen, then, as the advent of the freedom to spend and allocate time – which may or may not be welcomed.

A more general approach to time which we have introduced at several points relates to the importance of recognizing the beginnings, middles, and ends of situations and experiences and therefore the importance of pacing work with people during the process of moving through residential living. It is necessary to set realistic goals with clients which relate to the overall purpose of the worker's involvement – and a central aspect of this is the way the individual experiences time: whether he is ready to begin or to end (and whether in some sense events are 'early', or 'late'). This links directly to the stress that we have also placed on continuous connections through time. We have suggested on several occasions that it is necessary to be both backward-looking and forward-looking in helping people through the residential experience. In order to help people in the present it is often necessary to review, recall, or hold on to past events in their lives – whether it be protecting a child's favourite toys, allowing an old lady to reminisce about the good times in her life, or discussing the events that led up to an admission for psychiatric treatment. Similarly it is necessary to review and plan for the future in the ways we have described: the ability to cope with the pressures of the present may be very much bound up with plans and hopes for leaving.

Most importantly, time is a concept which relates closely to the idea of change. It is therefore at the basis of this entire discussion. We have tried to concentrate our attention on the positive aspects of change – on hope, expectations, and anticipations. This requires a view of the future and an ability to make predictions of what we expect to happen and what we hope may happen. Acting on the basis of predictions inevitably involves an element of risk-taking and as we indicated in the Introduction, risk-taking is an unavoidable part of the residential experience. There are few, if any, certain situations and we can only make informed guesses about likely outcomes. Helping people to leave care is therefore a process of identifying desirable outcomes and seeking ways of making those outcomes more likely – but in the knowledge that this necessarily involves taking risks.

These ideas about the importance of time can, of course, be considerably extended in relation to many different settings. We have introduced them here to illustrate and emphasize the fact that social work action and change in the residential setting should be seen not only in relation to organizational factors and individual needs but can also be seen in the wider frame of reference of the time and process elements which have been described both implicitly and explicitly throughout this book.

The process of leaving an enclosed living situation, like the process of admission to such an environment, involves action and change but it also involves making decisions. One of the most important issues which we feel emerges clearly from the book is the fact that the most appropriate decisions from the point of view of individuals are often substantially restricted by the institutional, organizational, and other systems within which they have to be made. It is, in other words, often not possible to make the best or most desirable decision because of attitudes, or because of inadequacy of resources. It is particularly significant that only in the case of children has it been possible for us to begin the discussion by assuming a ready acceptance of the proposition that social workers should and can play a major role in planning for leaving residential care. Only with children are existing practices and expectations such that social workers frequently become involved in the leaving process – and even with this group there is evidence that social work involvement leaves much to be desired.

We have, therefore, seen it as important to explore some of the policy issues which must be examined and developed if it is to become possible for social work practice to advance. The considerations are many and complex and clearly it is very different, for example, to describe the need for more varied resources and innovative practice to help older people back into the community, than to consider the nature of the social work role in helping people in the context of the multi-disciplinary team in a psychiatric hospital. Nevertheless, in each of the different contexts that we have discussed it is obvious that 'good decisions' about how best to help people can only be made in individual cases if resources are sufficiently extensive and varied and if attitudes are sufficiently positive to create and support a range of options.

For the individual, both admission and departure involve crossing boundaries in a variety of senses. In the most obvious sense a change of environment involves learning, or relearning the skills necessary to survive in the new environment. This inevitably leads to some degree of stress or anxiety and although it might be argued that this is essential to stimulate learning, it is important that social workers should recognize their role in helping to prevent anxiety becoming disabling or damaging. Such transitions also involve role and status change and this too will involve learning and adaptation. We have tried to show that, just as entry to an institution can be regarded as both distressing and as a relief or sanctuary, so departure can also frequently be characterized by feelings of ambivalence. Even those who eagerly look forward to release may experience disappointment, anxiety, or regret. For these and for the other reasons we have discussed we believe that there can be a very important role for social workers.

If departure can be seen as a boundary crossing for the resident, patient, or inmate then it can also be recognized as a boundary for social workers. As we have shown, it can be very difficult to clarify respective roles at these boundary points — whether it be the role of the hospital social worker versus that of the field social worker; prison welfare officer or probation officer; residential worker or field-worker. Our main purpose here has not been, other than in very general terms, to identify or clarify 'who does what?' since we believe that such decisions must be individualized. What is important is that different staff groups should work together, with clients, throughout the process of moving into, through, and out of residential living. In spite of the continuing debate about the respective roles of the residential and field social workers, there is broad, general agreement about the major focus of concern of each group and, at the boundary points, it should be possible to establish procedures for decision-making which will clarify the responsibility for action in individual situations. In concluding our previous book (Brearley *et al.* 1980) we stated our belief that:

'Many of the things that residential workers do involve social work skills, . . . It is essential that field and residential workers should be able to facilitate the continuing of social work help both during and after admission. Together they are able to offer a more informed service. Co-operation and collaboration are important to facilitate exchange and to ease the admission process: communication is important because it leads to an improved service for clients.'

(pp. 204–05)

We would wish to reiterate and stress this in the present context – with the insertion of the concept of leaving or departure as well as admission.

Finally, it is important to return to the concept of successful departure. This can mean many things and is likely to depend on a variety of factors – the original purpose of the placement and the extent to which the problems that led to the placement have been resolved which, in turn, is bound up with how far an individual can be described as being 'ready' to leave; the impact of the institution; the degree of practical and emotional preparation that has taken place; and the extent of the relationships that can be carried on in a supportive way after departure. In the preceding chapters we have set out primarily to demonstrate that social workers can play an important part in contributing to a successful outcome. The way in which people leave residential care is likely to have an important impact on their continuing experience and we have shown some of the ways in which social workers may help to create a more positive experience. Above all, it is essential that the outcomes of the

178 *Leaving Residential Care*

total residential experience should be related to the actions and experiences that take place throughout the process of moving through care: outcomes should be a planned result of careful decision-making and action, regularly reviewed with the client during the process. Departure can be viewed both as an event in one person's life, at a point in time and as a part of a continuing experience; in both senses it is an important event which demands more time and careful attention and action than has often been the case.

References

Adcock, M. (1981) The right of a child to a permanent placement. In M. Freeman, M. Adcock, and H. Bevan (eds) *Rights of Children*. BAAF 1981.

Adcock, M. and White, R. (1980) Care orders or the assumption of parental rights – the long-term effects. *Journal of Social Welfare Law* September: 257–64.

Age Concern England (1975) Manifesto on the place of the retired and the elderly in modern society. Age Concern.

Age Concern Greater London (1980) Discharge from hospital. The social worker's view.

Alexander, J. R. and Eldon, A. (1979) Characteristics of elderly people admitted to hospital. Part III, homes and sheltered housing. *Journal of Epidemiology and Community Health* **33** (March): 91–5.

Anthony, S. (1973) *The Discovery of Death in Childhood and After*. Harmondsworth: Penguin.

Arden, N. (1977) *Child of a System*. London: Quartet.

ABAFA (1976) The adopted persons need for information about his background. ABAFA pamphlet (revised edn).

—— (1977) Working with children who are joining new families.

—— (1979) Planning for children in long-term care.

Avon County Council, Social Services Department (1980) Admissions to homes for the elderly. A survey and assessment of alternatives.

Ayllon, T. and Azrin, N. H. (1968) *The Token Economy. A Motivational System for Therapy and Rehabilitation*. New York: Appleton-Century-Crofts.

Barton, R. (1959) *Institutional Neurosis*. Bristol: John Wright.

Bean, P. (1979) The Mental Health Act 1959: rethinking an old problem. *British Journal of Law and Society* **6** (1).

Bebbington, A. C. (1978) The elderly at home survey: changes in the provision of domiciliary social services to the elderly over fourteen years. University of Kent Personal Social Services Research Unit Discussion Paper No. 87.

Blenkner, M., Bloom, M., and Nielson, M. (1971) A research and demonstration project of protective services. *Social Casework* **52** (8): 483–99.

Bloom, C. V. (1968) *Children Are Our Concern*. Barnado School of Printing.

Bloom, M. and Blenkner, M. (1970) Assessing functioning of older persons living in the community. *The Gerontologist* 10 (pt 1): 31–7.

Booth, T. (1980) Measuring dependency. *Community Care*, 31 Jan. 1980, pp. 15–18.

Bosanquet, N. (1978) *A Future for Old Age.* London: Temple Smith/ New Society.

Bowlby, J. (1951) *Maternal Care and Mental Health.* World Health Organization.

Bradshaw, J. (1975) Research and the family fund. *Concern* 16: 28–32.

Braverman, A. and Baldock, P. (1980) An end to the old people's swop shop. *Social Work Today* 11 (45): 16–17.

Brearley, C. P. (1976) Old people in care. Supplement to *Community Care* 27 Oct. 1976.

—— (1977) *Residential Work with the Elderly.* London: Routledge and Kegan Paul.

Brearley, P., Hall, F., Gutridge, P., Jones, G., and Roberts, G. (1980) *Admission to Residential Care.* London: Tavistock Publications.

BASW (1977) Children in care: a BASW Charter of Rights. *Social Work Today* 8 (25): 7–9.

—— Special Interest Group on Ageing (1978) *A Happier Old Age.*

—— (1979) *Teamwork: For and Against. An Appraisal of Multi-disciplinary Practice.* BASW: Birmingham.

Britton, C. (1955) Casework techniques in the child care services. *Case Conference*, January 1955, pp. 3–15.

Brocklehurst, J. C. (1974) Old people in institutions – their rights. Age Concern England.

Brown, D. M. (1978) Kinloss Court Sheltered Housing Scheme. A report on the first year's monitoring. Hampshire County Council Social Services Dept.

Brown, G. W., Bone, M., Dalison, D., and Wing, J. K. (1966) *Schizophrenia and Social Care.* London, Oxford University Press.

Bucher, R. and Stelling, J. (1969) Characteristics of Professional Organization. *Journal of Health and Social Behaviour*, 10 (1): 3–15.

Burgess, C. (1981) *In Care and Into Work.* Tavistock Publications.

Burton, L. (1974) *Care of the Child Facing Death.* Routledge and Kegan Paul.

Butler, A. and Oldman, C. (1979) A question of choice. *New Age* 8 (Winter): 25–6.

Butler, A. W. J., Oldman, C. M., and Wright, R. M. A. (1979) Sheltered housing for the elderly: a critical review. University of Leeds Dept. of Social Policy and Administration Research Monograph.

Butler, R. N. (1963) The life review: an interpretation of reminiscence in the aged. *J. for the Study of Interpersonal Processes* 26 (1): 65–76.

Butterfield, E. and Baumeister, A. (eds) (1970) *Residential Facilities for the Mentally Retarded.* Chicago: Aldine Publishing Company.

Butterfield, E. C. and Zigler, E. (1968) The effects of differing institutional climates on the effectiveness of social reinforcement in the mentally retarded. *American Journal of Mental Deficiency* **72**: 815–27.

Carver, V. and Liddiard, P. (1978) *An Ageing Population*. London: Hodder and Stoughton.

CCETSW (1973) Residential work is part of social work. CCETSW Paper 3.

Central Health Services Council (1959) Report of the Committee on the Welfare of Children in Hospital. (Chairman: Platt.) London: HMSO.

–––– (1967) Report of a Sub-Committee of the Standing Medical Advisory Committee on Child Welfare Centres. (Chairman: Sir Wilfred Sheldon.) London: HMSO.

Central Statistical Office (1981) *Social Trends II*. London: HMSO.

Challis, D. and Davies, B. (1980) A new approach to community care for the elderly. *British Journal of Social Work* **10**: 1–18.

Coleman, J. C. (1980) *The Nature of Adolescence*. London: Methuen.

Collins, M. and Collins, D. (1975) *Kith and Kids*. Human Horizons Series. London: Souvenir Press.

Cooper, D. (1972) *The Death of the Family*. Harmondsworth: Pelican.

Corden, J., Kuipers, J., and Wilson, K. (1978) After prison. Papers in Community Studies No. 21. Dept. of Soc. Admin. and Social Work, University of York.

Creer, C. and Wing, J. K. (1974) *Schizophrenia at Home*. Surbiton: National Schizophrenia Fellowship.

Crompton, M. (1980) *Respecting Children. Social Work with Young People*. London: Arnold.

Davies, B. (1981) Strategic goals and piecemeal innovations: adjusting to the new balance of needs and resources. In E. M. Goldberg and S. Hatch (eds) *A New Look at the Personal Social Services*. Policy Studies Institute Discussion Paper No. 4.

Davies, B. and Knapp, M. (1981) *Old People's Homes and the Production of Welfare*. London: Routledge and Kegan Paul Library of Social Work.

Davies, M. (1979) Swopping the Old Around. *Community Care*, 18 Oct. 1979, pp. 16–17.

Day, C. (1980) Access to birth records – the impact of Section 26 of the Children Act 1975. ABAFA.

Department of Education and Science (1978) Report of the Committee of Enquiry into the Education of Handicapped Children and Young People. (Chairman: Mary Warnock.) London: HMSO.

DHSS and the Welsh Office (1971) Better services for the mentally handicapped. Cmnd. 4683. London: HMSO.

_____ _____ (1978) A happier old age. A discussion document on elderly people in our society. London: HMSO.

_____ (1969) Report of the Committee of Enquiry into Allegations of Ill-Treatment of Patients and Other Irregularities at the Ely Hospital, Cardiff. Cmnd. 3957. London: HMSO.

_____ (1972a) Report of the Committee on Nursing. (Chairman: Asa Briggs.) Cmnd. 5115. London: HMSO.

_____ (1972b) Statistical and Research Report Series No. 3. London: HMSO.

_____ (1975) Better services for the mentally ill. Cmnd. 6233. London: HMSO.

_____ (1976a) Foster care: a guide to practice. London: HMSO.

_____ (1976b) Report of the Committee on Child Health Services. (Chairman: S. D. M. Court.) *Fit for the Future.* London: HMSO.

_____ (1977) Mentally handicapped children: a plan for action. National Development Group Pamphlet No. 2. London: HMSO.

_____ (1978a) Health and personal social service statistics for England. London: HMSO.

_____ (1978b) Review of the Mental Health Act. London: HMSO.

_____ (1979a) Report of the Committee of Enquiry into Mental Handicap Nursing and Care. (Chairman: Peggy Jay.) London: HMSO.

_____ (1979b) Residential care for the elderly in London.

_____ (1981a) Care in action. A handbook of policies and priorities for the health and personal social services in England. London: HMSO.

_____ (1981b) Care in the community. A consultative document on moving resources for care. London: HMSO.

DHSS/Scottish, Welsh and Northern Ireland Offices (1981) Growing older. Cmnd. 8173. London: HMSO.

Dingwell, A. (1980) Problems of team work in primary care. In S. Lonsdale, A. Webb, and T. L. Briggs (eds) *Teamwork in the Personal Social Services and Health Care.* pp. 111–37. London: Croom Helm.

The Disability Alliance (1979) The government's failure to plan for disablement in old age. London: Disability Alliance.

Drillien, C. and Drummond, M. (eds) (1977) *Neurodevelopmental Problems in Early Childhood.* Oxford: Blackwell Scientific Publications.

Early, D. (1965) Industrial and social rehabilitation. In H. Freeman and J. Farndale (eds) *New Aspects of the Mental Health Services.* London: Pergamon Press, pp. 149–52.

Elliott, J. R. (1975) Living in hospital. The social needs of people in long-term care. King Edwards Hospital Fund for London.

Ennals, D. (1978) The role of residential care. *Social Work Today* **10** (7): 14–15.

Erikson, E. H. (1965) *Childhood and Society.* Harmondsworth: Pelican.

Evers, H. K. (1981) Multidisciplinary teams in geriatric wards. Myth or reality? Dept. of Sociology, University of Warwick.

Fairhurst, E. (1977) Teamwork as panacea: some underlying assumptions. Geigy Unit for Research in Ageing, University of Manchester.

Fairweather, G. W., Sanders, D. H., Maynard, H., Cressler, D. C., and Black, D. S. (1969) *Community Life for the Mentally Ill.* Chicago Ill.: Aldine.

Fanshawe, E. (1975) *Rachel.* London: Bodley Head.

Fanshel, D. and Shinn, E. (1978) *Children in Foster Care: A Longitudinal Study.* New York: Columbia UP.

Farrington, D. S., Shelton, W., and McKay, V. R. (1968) Observations on runaway children from a residential setting. In R. J. N. Tod (ed.) *Disturbed Children.* London: Longman.

Ferlic, E. (1980) Directory of initiatives in the community care of the elderly. University of Kent PSSRU.

Foster, J. and Remfry, P. (1981) The elderly in the community. A study of people aged 65 and over living in North Tyneside in 1979. North Tyneside Metropolitan Borough. Social Services Dept.

Fox, A. M. (1974) They get this training, but they don't really know how you feel. National Bureau for Research into Crippling Diseases. London: Action Research.

Fraiberg, S. (1959) *The Magic Years.* London: Methuen.

Gath, A. (1978) *Down's Syndrome and the Family: The Early Years.* London: Academic Press.

Godek, S. (1977) Leaving care. Barnado Social Work Papers No. 2.

Goffman, E. (1961) *Asylums. Essays on the Social Situation of Mental Patients and Other Inmates.* New York: Anchor Books, Doubleday.

Goldie, N. (1977) The division of labour among the mental health professions — a negotiated or imposed order? In M. Stacey (ed.) *Health and the Division of Labour.* London: Croom Helm.

Goss, M. E. W. (1963) Patterns of bureaucracy among hospital staff physicians. In Friedson, E. (ed.) *The Hospital in Modern Society.* New York: Free Press.

Gostin, L. and Rassaby, E. (1980) *Representing the Mentally Ill and Handicapped.* Sunbury, Middlesex: Quatermaine House.

Gray, B. and Isaacs, B. (1979) *Care of the Elderly Mentally Infirm.* London: Tavistock Publications.

Gray, M. (1980a) For the good of their health. *Social Work Today,* 8 July, pp. 10–11.

—— (1980b) Section 47 — life or liberty. *New Age* 11 (Summer): 22–5.

Gregory, S. (1976) *The Deaf Child and His Family.* London: George Allen and Unwin.

Gunzberg, H. (1970) The Hospital as a normalizing training environment. *Journal of Mental Subnormality* 31 (Dec.): 71–83.

Gutridge, P. (1970) The group. *Barnado Forum*: 120–24.
―――― (1980) Admission and children. In P. Brearley *et al. Admission to Residential Care*. London: Tavistock Publications.

Hallett, C. and Stevenson, O. (1980) *Child Abuse: Aspects of Interprofessional Cooperation*. London: George Allen and Unwin.
Hannam, C. (1975) *Parents and Mentally Handicapped Children*. London: Penguin/MIND.
Harris, A. I. (1968) *Social Welfare for the Elderly*. London: HMSO.
Hart, T. (1977) *Safe on a Seesaw*. London: Quartet.
HMSO (1957) Report of the Royal Commission on the Law Relating to Mental Illness and Mental Deficiency. Cmnd. 169. London.
Hewett, S. (1970) *The Family and the Handicapped Child*. London: Allen and Unwin.
Hewett, S., Ryan, P., and Wing, J. K. (1975) Living without the mental hospitals. *Journal of Social Policy* 4: 391–404.
Hitchman, J. (1966) *The King of the Barbareens*. London: Peacock.
Hoggett, B. (1976) *Social Work and the Law: Mental Health*. London: Sweet and Maxwell.
―――― (1981) *Social Work and the Law: Parents and Children*. London: Sweet and Maxwell.
Hudson, B. L. (1978) Behavioural social work with schizophrenic patients in the community. *British Journal of Social Work* 8 (2): 159–70.

James, L. and Bytheway, B. (1978) Is sheltered housing an alternative to part III? Medical Sociology Unit, University of Swansea.
Jeffree, D. and McConkey, R. (1977) *Let Me Speak; Let Me Play; Teaching the Handicapped Child*. Human Horizons Series. London: Souvenir Press.
Jehu, D. (1963) Casework before admission to care. ACCO, Monograph 1.
Jones, G. (1980) The decision to admit: policy framework and practice. In P. Bearley *et al. Admission to Residential Care*. London: Tavistock Publications.
Jones, K. (1979) Integration or disintegration of the mental health service: some reflections on developments in Britain since the 1950s. In M. Meacher (ed.) *New Methods of Mental Health Care*. London: Mental Health Foundation, pp. 3–14.
Jones, M. (1968) *Social Psychiatry in Practice*. Harmondsworth: Penguin.
―――― (1974) Psychiatry, systems theory, education and change. *British Journal of Psychiatry* 124: 75–80.
Jones, W. (1970) Keeping the memories of childhood. *Social Work Today* 1 (5): 22–3.

Kahan, B. (1979) *Growing up in Care — 10 people talking*. Oxford: Basil Blackwell.

Kay, N. (1980) Letter to *Community Care*, 15 Feb. 1980, pp. 11–12.

Kew, S. (1976) *Handicap and the Family Crisis — A Study of the Siblings of Handicapped Children*. London: Pitman.

King, R., Raynes, N., and Tizard, J. (1971) *Patterns of Residential Care*. London: Routledge and Kegan Paul.

Kirman, B. (1951) The backward baby. *Journal of Mental Science* **99**: 531–41.

—— (1972) *The Mentally Handicapped Child*. London: Institute for Research into Mental and Multiple Handicap.

Kushlick, A. (1970) Residential care for the mentally subnormal. *Journal of the Royal Society of Health* **90** (5): 71–83.

La Barre, W. (1969) Adolescence: a crucible of change. *Social Casework*, Jan. 1969, pp. 22–6.

Lamb, R. H. and Associates (1971) *Rehabilitation in Community Mental Health*. London: Jossey-Bass.

Larsen, H. (1976) *Don't Forget Tom*. New York: Crowell.

Lasson, I. (1981) *Where's My Mum?* Birmingham: Pepar Publications.

Lawton, M. P. (1980) *Environment and Aging*. Monterey: Brooks/Cole Publishing.

Leach, J. and Wing, J. K. (1978) The effectiveness of a service for helping destitute men. *British Journal of Psychiatry* **133**: 481–92.

Lee, P. and Pithers, D. (1980) Radical residential child care — Trojan horse or non-runner? In M. Brake and R. Bailey (eds) *Radical Social Work and Practice*. London: Arnold.

Leeming, J. T. (1979) Rehabilitation: Unit 11, An Ageing Population Course. Open University.

Liberman, R. P. (1971) Behaviour modification with chronic mental patients. *Journal of Chronic Disability* **23**: 803–12.

Lieberman, M. A. (1974) Symposium — long term care: research policy and practice. Relocation research and social policy. *Gerontologist* **14** (6): 494–500.

Lonsdale, G., Elfer, P., and Ballard, R. (1979) *Children, Grief and Social Work*. Oxford: Basil Blackwell.

Lonsdale, S., Webb, A. L., and Briggs, T. L. (1980) *Teamwork in the Personal Social Services and Health Care*. London: Croom Helm.

Lowy, L. (1979) *Social Work with the Aging*. New York: Harper and Row.

McClean, J. D. (1981) *The Legal Context of Social Work*. London: Butterworth.

Mann, S. and Cree, W. (1976) 'New' long-stay psychiatric patients: a national survey of fifteen mental hospitals in England and Wales 1972/3. *Psychological Medicine* **6**: 603–06.

Marris, P. (1974) *Loss and Change*. London: Routledge and Kegan Paul.
Marx, I. M., Connolly, J., Hallam, R., and Phillpott, R. (1975) Nurse therapists in behavioural psychotherapy. *British Medical Journal* 3: 144–48.
Meacher, M. (ed.) (1979) *New Methods of Mental Health Care*. London: Mental Health Foundation, Pergamon.
Miller, L. (1979) Toward a classification of aging behaviour. *Gerontologist* 19 (3): 283–90.
MIND (1977) MIND's Evidence to the Royal Commission on the NHS with regard to services for mentally ill people. London: MIND.
Ministry of Health (1962) Hospital plan for England and Wales, 1962. Cmnd. 1604. London: HMSO.
—— (1967) *Child Welfare Centres*. London: HMSO.
Minor, W. W. and Courlander, M. (1979) The post-release trauma thesis. A reconsideration of the risk of early parole failure. *J. of Research in Crime and Delinquency* 16 (2): 273–93.
Morris, P. (1969) *Put Away: A Sociological Study of Institutions for the Mentally Retarded.* London: Routledge and Kegan Paul.
Mulvey, T. (1977–78) After care – who cares. Concern. *Journal of National Children's Bureau* no. 26 (Winter): 26–30.

NACRO (1980) *Helping the Homeless*.
National Children's Bureau (1970) *Living with Handicap*. Younghusband *et al.* (eds). London: National Children's Bureau.
National Secular Society (1971) *The Rights of Old People*. London: National Secular Society.
Norman, A. J. (1979) Rights and risk. A discussion document on civil liberty in old age. London: NCCOP.

Ollivant, B. (1979) Rights on discharge. In D. Harris and J. Hyland (eds) *Rights in Residence*. London: Residential Care Assoc.
Olsen, R. (ed.) (1976) Differential approaches in social work with the mentally disordered. Birmingham: British Association of Social Workers.
—— (ed.) (1979) The care of the mentally disordered. Birmingham: British Association of Social Workers.
O'Neill, T. (1981) *A Place Called Hope*. Oxford: Basil Blackwell.
Oswin, M. (1971) *The Empty Hours: A Study of Weekend Life of Handicapped Children in Institutions*. London: Allen Lane.
—— (1978) *Children Living in Long-Stay Hospitals*. Spastics International Medical Publications. London: Heinemann Medical Books.

Page, R. and Clark, G. A. (eds) (1977) *Who Cares? Young People in Care Speak Out*. National Children's Bureau, Northbourne Press.
Park, C. C. (1967) *The Siege*. Harmondsworth: Penguin.

Parker, R. A. (1980) *Caring for Separated Children*. London: National Children's Bureau, Macmillan.

Parker, R. (1981) Tending and social policy. In E. M. Goldberg and S. Hatch (eds) *A New Look at the Personal Social Services*. Policy Studies Institute Discussion Paper No. 4.

Pattie, A. H. and Gilleard, C. J. (1979) *Clifton Assessment Procedures for the Elderly*. London: Hodder and Stoughton.

Payne, C. (1979) You are going to find it tough when you leave care. In G. E. Barritt (ed.) *Rehabilitating the Child in Care*. National Children's Homes Occasional Paper No. 2.

Personal Social Services Council (1977) *Residential Care Reviewed*.

―――― (1980) *Catalogue of Development in the Care of Old People*.

Pharis, M. E. (1967) The use of adolescents' creative writing in diagnosis and treatment. *Social Casework*, Feb. 1969, pp. 67–74.

Plank, D. (1977) Caring for the elderly: report of a study of various means of caring for dependent elderly people in 8 London boroughs. London: Greater London Council.

―――― (1978a) Old people's homes are NOT the last refuge. *Community Care*, 1 Mar. 1978, pp. 16–18.

―――― (1978b) The policy context. Paper given to PSSRU/PSSC conference on evaluating new domiciliary and day interventions for the elderly.

Pless, I. and Pinkerton, P. (1975) *Chronic Childhood Disorder – Promoting Patterns of Adjustment*. London: Henry Kimpton.

Pope, P. (1980) Emergency admissions into homes for the elderly. *Social Work Service* no. 24, Sept. 1980, pp. 18–22.

Pringle, M. L. K. (1975) *The Needs of Children*. London: Hutchinson.

Raphael, W. and Peers, V. (1972) *Psychiatric Hospitals Viewed by Their Patients*. London: King Edward's Hospital Fund.

Rayner, E. (1971) *Human Development*. London: Allen and Unwin.

Reid, H. (1979) From care to independence. In Barnado Publications *In the Year of the Child – Barnado Child Care Services*.

RCA/BASW (1976) How can residential and field social workers cooperate? *Social Work Today* 7 (12): 346–48.

―――― (1978) The key worker – the respective and reciprocal roles of residential and field social workers. In RCA Review *Heads and Hearts*. Residential Care Association.

Reynolds, D. (1980) Closing homes 'to help the elderly'. *Community Care*, 3 July 1980, pp. 20–3.

Righton, P. (1970) Co-operation between community-based social workers and residential staff. Keele University.

―――― (1973) A continuum of care. The link between field and residential work. Barnado Lecture 1973.

Roberts, Gwyneth (1981) *Essential Law for Social Workers*. London: Oyez.

Roberts, J. A. (1981) An evaluation of the Amblecote House Project –
assessment and short-stay for the elderly. Dudley Social Services Dept.
Rowbottom, R. and Hey, A. (1978) Organization of services for the
mentally ill. A Working Paper BIOSS. London: Brunel University.
Rowe, J. and Lambert, L. (1973) Children who wait: a study of
children needing substitute families. ABAA.
Rowlett, C. and Dews, E. (1979) The story of Billy. *Social Work Today*
11 (9): 16–18.
Rowlings, C. (1978) Social work with the elderly: some problems and
possibilities. University of Keele Social Work Research Project.
_____ (1981) *Social Work with Elderly People*. London: George Allen
and Unwin.
Royal College of Psychiatrists (1980) Report of the Working Party on
Rehabilitation. *Psychiatric Rehabilitation in the 1980s*. London:
Royal College of Psychiatrists.
Russell, P. (1978) *The Wheelchair Child*. Human Horizons Series.
London: Souvenir Press.
Russian, R-B. (1975) Idealisation during adolescence. Smith College
Studies in Social Work, June 1975, pp. 211–29.
Rutter, M. (1972) *Maternal Deprivation Reassessed*. Harmondsworth:
Penguin.

Sayer, P., Forbes, D., Newman, P., and Jameson, T. (1976) Positive
planning for children in care. *Social Work Today* 8 (2): 9–11.
Scheff, T. J. (1966) *Being Mentally Ill*. London: Weidenfield and
Nicolson.
Schiphorst, B. (1979) Development of a functional rating chart for the
elderly: application in Cleveland and Sunderland Social Services
Departments. *Social Work Service* no. 19 (March): 3–10.
Scull, A. T. (1977) *Decarceration*. New York: Random House.
Sereny, G. (1974) *The Case of Mary Bell*. London: Arrow Books.
Shaw, I. and Walton, R. (1979) Transition to residence in homes for
elderly. In D. Harris and J. Hyland (eds) *Rights in Residence*.
Residential Care Association.
Shaw, M. and Lebens, K. (1978) *Substitute Family Care*. Vol. II *What
Shall We Do with the Children?* London: ABAFA.
Siegler, M. and Osmond, H. (1966) Models of madness. *British Journal
of Psychiatry* 112 (1): 193–203.
Siegler, M. and Osmond, H. (1971) Goffman's model of mental illness.
British Journal of Psychiatry 119: 419–24.
Slack, G. and Gibbins, J. (1979) *Organising After Care*. National
Corporation for the Care of Old People.
Slasberg, C. and Godek, S. (1980) A working relationship. *Social Work
Today* 12 (6): 12–14.
Smaldino, A. (1975) The importance of hope in the casework relation-
ship. *Social Casework* 56 (6): 328–33.

Smith, G. (1970) *Social Work and the Sociology of Organizations.* London: Routledge and Kegan Paul.
Smith, H. L. (1958) Two lines of authority: the hospitals dilemma. In E. G. Jaco (ed.) *Patients, Physicians and Illness: Source Book in Behavioural Science and Medicine.* Glencoe, Ill.: Free Press.
Socialist Child Care Collective (1975) *Changing Child Care: Cuba, China and the Challenging of Our Values.* London: Writers and Readers Publishing Co-operative.
Specht, H. and Vickery, A. (1977) *Integrating Social Work Methods.* London: Allen and Unwin.
Stevenson, O. and Parsloe, P. (1978) *Social Service Teams: The Practitioners View.* London: HMSO.
Stoeffler, V. R. (1972) The separation phenomena in residential treatment. In J. K. Whittaker and A. E. Trieschman (eds) *Children Away from Home – A Source Book of Residential Treatment.* London: Aldine, 1972.
Stone, J. and Taylor, F. (1977) *Handbook for Parents with a Handicapped Child.* London: Arrow Books.
Stroud, J. (1963) *On the Loose.* Harmondsworth: Penguin.

Tarran, E. (1981) Parents' views of medical and social work services for families with young cerebral-palsied children. *Dev. Medicine and Child Neurology* 23 (2): 173.
Thomas, L. (1967) *This Time Next Week.* London: Pan Books.
Thornton, P. and Moore, J. (1980) The placement of elderly people in private households: an analysis of current provisions. The University of Leeds Dept. of Social Policy and Administration Monograph.
Timms, N. (1972) *Recording in Social Work.* London: Routledge and Kegan Paul.
—— (1973) *The Receiving End – Consumer Accounts of Social Help for Children.* London: Routledge and Kegan Paul.
Tinker, A. (1980) Housing the elderly near relatives. Moving and other options. Dept. of the Environment. London: HMSO.
Tizard, B. (1977) *Adoption: A Second Chance.* London: Open Books.
Tizard, J. (1964) *Community Services for the Mentally Handicapped.* London: Oxford University Press.
Tobin, S. S. and Liebermann, M. A. (1976) *Last Home for the Aged.* California: Jossey-Bass.
Townsend, P. (1962) *The Last Refuge.* London: Routledge and Kegan Paul.
—— (1973) *The Social Minority.* London: Allen Lane.
—— (1976) The sociology of ageing: residential homes and institutions. In *Old Age Today and Tomorrow.* British Association for the Advancement of Science.
Townsend, P. and Wedderburn, D. (1965) *The Aged in the Welfare State.* London: Bell.

Toy Libraries Association (1975) *Toys for Children with Speech, Hearing and Language Difficulties* and *Toys and Activities for Handicapped Children*. Potters Bar: Toy Libraries Association.

Triseliotis, J. (1980) *New Developments in Foster Care and Adoption*. London: Routledge and Kegan Paul.

Vinter, R. D. (1963) Analysis of treatment organizations. *Social Work* 8 (3): 3–15. New York: NASW.

Vorrath, H. H. and Brendtro, B. K. (1974) *Positive Peer Culture*. Aldine.

Walmsley, R. (1972) *Steps from Prison*. Inner London Probation and After Care Service.

Ward, L. (1980) The social work task. In R. G. Walton and D. Elliott (eds) *Residential Care*. Oxford: Pergamon.

Ward, P. (1980) *Quality of Life in Residential Care*. Personal Social Services Council.

Wardle, M. (1975) Hippopotamus or cow? On not communicating about children. *Social Work Today* 6 (14): 430–32.

Webb, A. L. and Hobdell, M. (1980) Co-ordination and teamwork in the health and personal social services. In S. Lonsdale, A. Webb and T. L. Briggs (eds) *Teamwork in the Personal Social Services and Health Care*, pp. 97–110. London: Croom Helm.

Wendelken, C. (1981) The search for identity. *Social Work Today* 12 (19): 8–10.

White, K. J. (1980) Respect for the person in community. In D. Lane and K. White (eds) *Why Care?* RCA Annual Review.

Wilkin, D. (1979) *Caring for the Mentally Handicapped*. London: Croom Helm.

Wilkin, D. and Jolley, D. (1979) Behavioral Problems Among Old People in Geriatric Wards, Psychogeriatric Wards and Residential Homes 1976–78. Univ. of Manchester Depts. of Psychiatry and Community Medicine Research Report No. 1.

Wilks, J. and Wilks, E. (1974) *Bernard, bringing up our mongol son*. Routledge and Kegan Paul.

Williams, I. (1979) *The Care of the Elderly in the Community*. London: Croom Helm.

Wills, W. D. (1970) *A Place Like Home. A Pioneer Hostel for Boys*. NISWT Series No. 17. London: George Allen and Unwin.

Wing, J. K. and Brown, G. W. (1970) *Institutionalism and Schizophrenia*. London: Cambridge University Press.

Wing, J. K. and Olsen, R. (eds) (1979) *Community Care for the Mentally Disabled*. London: Oxford Univ. Press.

Winnicott, C. (1964) *Child Care and Social Work*. Bookstall Publications.

Wood, K. (1979) Towards independence. A study of adolescents in care. Church of England Children's Society. Study Paper No. 4.

Woodburn, M. (1975) *The Social Implications of Spina Bifida*. London: National Foundation for Educational Research.

Yawney, B. A. and Slover, D. L. (1973) Relocation of the elderly. *Social Work* **18** (3): 86–95.

Younghusband, E., Birchall, D., Davie, R., and Pringle, M. L. K. (eds) (1970) *Living With Handicap*. London: National Children's Bureau.

Name Index

Adcock, M., 44, 67, 179
Age Concern England, 128, 179
Age Concern Greater London,
  142, 179
Alexander, J. R., 124, 179
Anthony, S., 64, 179
Arden, N., 67, 179
ABAFA, 67, 76, 79, 179
Avon County Council, 134, 179
Ayllon, T., 155, 179
Azrin, N. H., 155, 179

Baldock, P., 23, 180
Ballard, R., 64, 185
Barritt, G. E., 187
Barton, R., 122, 131, 179
Baumeister, A., 100, 180
Bean, P., 46, 179
Bebbington, A. C., 118, 125, 179
Bevan, H., 179
Birchall, D., 191
Black, D. S., 183
Blenkner, M., 130, 136, 179
Bloom, C. V., 65, 89, 179
Bloom, M., 130, 136, 179, 180
Bone, M., 180
Booth, T., 124, 137, 180
Bosanquet, N., 119, 180
Bowlby, J., 19, 180
Bradshaw, J., 95, 180
Braverman, A., 23, 180
Brearley, C. P., 3, 9, 15, 28, 54,
  117, 123, 129, 138, 177, 180
Brendtro, B. K., 90, 190
Briggs, T. L., 24, 182, 185
BASW, 27, 28, 66, 79, 104, 119,
  156, 180

Britton, C., 80, 180
Brocklehurst, J. C., 131, 180
Brown, D. M., 126, 180
Brown, G. W., 152, 166, 180
Bucher, R., 158, 180
Burgess, C., 21, 180
Burton, L., 64, 102, 180
Butler, A. W. J., 123, 126, 131,
  180
Butler, R. N., 136, 180
Butterfield, E. C., 100, 180, 181
Bytheway, B., 125, 184

Carver, V., 140, 181
CCETSW, 26, 181
Central Health Services Council,
  97, 181
Central Statistical Office, 5, 7,
  181
Challis, D., 115, 141, 181
Clark, G. A., 65, 69, 73–4, 81,
  83, 84, 186
Coleman, J. C., 90, 181
Collins, D., 102, 181
Collins, M., 102, 181
Connolly, J., 186
Cooper, D., 86, 181
Courlander, M., 33, 186
Corden, J., 12, 22, 181
Cree, W., 148, 185
Creer, C., 148, 181
Cressler, D. C., 183
Crompton, M., 71, 181

Dalison, D., 180
Davie, R., 191

Davies, B., 17, 115, 126–27, 139, 141, 181
Davies, M., 131, 181
Day, C., 76, 181
Department of Education and Science, 100, 181
DHSS, 6, 7, 8, 45, 46, 47, 49, 67, 76, 94, 95, 97, 98, 99, 101, 123, 124, 147, 148, 150, 156, 163, 181
Dews, E., 21, 188
Dingwell, A., 157, 181
Disability Alliance, 122, 182
Drillien, C., 94, 182
Drummond, M., 94, 182

Early, D., 166, 182
Eldon, A., 124, 179
Elfer, P., 64, 185
Elliott, J. R., 131, 182
Ennals, D., 8, 182
Erikson, E. H., 90, 182
Evers, H. K., 25, 183

Fairhurst, E., 25, 140, 183
Fairweather, G. W., 170, 183
Fanshawe, E., 102, 183
Fanshel, D., 67, 183
Farrington, D. S., 86, 183
Ferlie, E., 126, 183
Forbes, D., 188
Foster, J., 123, 183
Fox, A. M., 102, 183
Fraiberg, S., 63, 183
Freeman, M., 179
Friedson, E., 183

Gath, A., 102, 183
Gibbins, J., 143–44, 188
Gilleard, C. J., 137, 187
Godek, S., 13–14, 18, 21, 26, 31, 32, 77, 89, 183
Goffman, E., 14, 122, 131, 151–52, 183
Goldberg, E. M., 187
Goldie, N., 154, 155, 156–57, 183

Goss, M. E. W., 154, 183
Gostin, L., 45, 52, 183
Gray, B., 141, 183
Gray, M., 54, 131, 183
Gregory, S., 102, 183
Gunsberg, H., 103, 183
Gutridge, P., 63, 76, 89, 90, 180, 184

Hall, F., 180
Hallam, R., 186
Hallett, C., 25, 184
Hannam, C., 102, 184
Harris, A. I., 122, 184
Hart, T., 86, 184
Hatch, S., 187
HMSO, 147, 184
Hewett, S., 102, 148, 184
Hey, A., 158, 188
Hitchman, J., 65, 69, 184
Hobdell, M., 158, 190
Hoggett, B., 54, 184
Hudson, B. L., 155, 184

Isaacs, B., 141, 183

Jaco, E. G., 189
James, L., 125, 184
Jameson, T., 188
Jeffree, D., 102, 184
Jehu, D., 67, 184
Jolley, D., 123, 190
Jones, G., 118, 180, 184
Jones, K., 149, 184
Jones, M., 155, 184
Jones, W., 78, 184

Kahan, B., 86, 185
Kay, N., 124, 185
Kew, S., 102, 185
King, R., 100, 152, 185
Kirman, B., 94, 102, 115, 185
Klaber, M., 100
Knapp, M., 17, 139, 181
Kuipers, J., 181
Kushlick, A., 99, 103, 185

La Barre, W., 90, 185
Lamb, R. H., 170, 185
Lambert, L., 67, 188
Larsen, H., 102, 185
Lasson, I., 76, 77, 87, 93, 185
Lawton, M. P., 137, 185
Leach, J., 148, 185
Lebens, K., 67, 188
Lee, P., 81–2, 185
Leeming, J. T., 139, 185
Liberman, R. P., 155, 185
Liddiard, P., 140, 181
Lieberman, M. A., 122, 130, 138, 185
Lonsdale, G., 64, 185
Lonsdale, S., 24, 182, 185
Lowy, L., 140, 185

McKay, V. R., 183
McClean, J. D., 54, 185
McConkey, R., 102, 184
Mann, S., 148, 185
Marris, P., 20, 186
Marx, I. M., 155, 186
Maynard, H., 183
Meacher, M., 163, 184, 186
Miller, L., 135, 186
Minahan, A., 107
MIND, 104, 150, 186
Ministry of Health, 99, 147, 186
Minor, W. W., 33, 186
Mitchell, R. G., 94, 95
Mittler, P., 98–9
Moore, J., 142, 189
Morris, P., 97, 186
Mulvey, T., 13, 20, 21, 26–7, 186

NACRO, 21, 186
National Secular Society, 129, 186
Newman, P., 188
Nielson, M., 130, 179
Norman, A. J., 130, 186

Oldman, C. M., 123, 126, 131, 180

Ollivant, B., 11, 13, 65, 186
Olsen, R., 166, 186
O'Neill, T., 65, 69, 78, 186
Osmond, H., 152, 155, 188
Oswin, M., 97, 99, 186

Page, R., 65, 69, 73–4, 81, 84, 186
Park, C. C., 102, 186
Parker, R. A., 65, 128, 187
Parsloe, P., 155, 189
Pattie, A. H., 137, 186
Payne, C., 16–17, 18, 25, 26–7, 64, 65, 67, 186
Peers, V., 170, 187
Personal Social Services Council 126, 131, 186
Pharis, M. E., 79, 187
Phillpott, R., 186
Pincus, A., 107
Pinkerton, P., 94, 187
Pithers, D., 81–2, 185
Plank, D., 22, 121, 124–25, 126, 187
Pless, I., 94, 187
Pope, P., 133, 187
Pringle, M. L. K., 66, 187, 191

Raphael, W., 170, 187
Rassaby, E., 45, 52, 183
Rayner, E., 90, 187
Raynes, N., 100, 152, 185
Reid, H., 65, 89, 90, 187
Remfry, P., 123, 183
Residential Care Association, 27 66, 79, 187
Reynolds, D., 123, 187
Righton, P., 26, 107, 187
Roberts, G., 54, 180, 187
Roberts, J. A., 139, 188
Rowbottom, R., 158, 188
Rowe, J., 67, 188
Rowlett, C., 21, 188
Rowlings, C., 140, 188
Royal College of Psychiatrists, 148. 156. 166. 170. 188

Russell, P., 102, 188
Russian, R. B., 90, 188
Rutter, M., 19, 188
Ryan, P., 148, 184

Sanders, D. H., 183
Sayer, P., 30, 188
Scheff, T. J., 151, 188
Schiphorst, B., 137, 188
Scull, A. T., 125, 188
Sereny, G., 67, 188
Shaw, I., 122, 188
Shaw, M., 67, 188
Shelton, W., 183
Shinn, E., 67, 183
Siegler, M., 152, 155, 188
Slack, G., 143–44, 188
Slasberg, C., 26, 188
Slover, D. L., 136, 191
Smaldino, A., 90, 188
Smith, G., 152, 189
Smith, H. L., 154, 189
Socialist Child Care Collective, 82, 189
Specht, H., 107, 189
Stacey, M., 183
Stelling, J., 155, 180
Stevenson, O., 25, 155, 189
Stoeffler, V. R., 70, 189
Stone, J., 102, 189
Stroud, J., 68, 189

Tarran, E., 102, 189
Taylor, F., 102, 189
Thomas, L., 11–12, 65, 85, 87, 189
Thornton, P., 142, 189
Timms, N., 69, 80, 189
Tinker, A., 142, 189
Tizard, B., 65, 189

Tizard, J., 97, 100, 152, 189
Tobin, S. S., 122, 138, 189
Townsend, P., 98, 121, 123, 125, 189
Toy Libraries Association, 102, 190
Trieschman, A. E., 189
Triseliotis, J., 76, 190

Vickery, A., 107, 189
Vinter, R. D., 153, 190
Vorrath, H. H., 90, 190

Walmsley, R., 22, 190
Walton, R., 122, 188
Ward, L., 60–1, 190
Ward, P., 123, 190
Wardle, M., 73, 190
Webb, A. L., 24, 158, 182, 190
Wedderburn, D., 125, 189
Wendelken, C., 20, 190
White, K. J., 88, 190
White, R., 44, 179
Whittaker, J. K., 189
Wilkin, D., 102, 123, 190
Wilks, E., 102, 190
Wilks, J., 102, 190
Williams, I., 135, 190
Wills, W. D., 17–18, 82, 190
Wilson, K., 181
Wing, J. K., 148, 166, 190
Winnicott, C., 80, 190
Wood, K., 21, 191
Woodburn, M., 102, 191
Wright, R. M. A., 123, 126, 180

Yawney, B. A., 136, 191
Younghusband, E., 94, 95, 191

Zigler, E., 100, 181

Subject Index

accommodation, 31, 91, 124–26, 129, 141–43
acute admission ward, 163
adaptation, 176
admission, 3–4, 25, 29; and children, 63–4, 66, 73, 93; and handicapped children, 96, 102, 104–09, 114–16; and elderly, 130–31
adolescence, 13–14, 21, 65, 70, 90
adoption, 64, 67, 87, 89, 92
advocate, 83
after care, 32–3; and children, 66, 88, 90, 91; and handicapped children, 107, 109, 114–15; and mentally ill, 158, 162–63
ambivalence, 12, 16, 66, 68, 70, 71, 72
apathy, 122
assessment, 30; and handicapped children, 99, 108; and elderly, 28, 119, 133–39, 144–45; and mentally ill, 160, 161, 164, 167, 168

Barnardo's Homes, 13–14, 65
behaviour, 85, 111, 112, 114, 135–36
behaviour modification, 109, 111, 114, 155
Better Services for the Mentally Handicapped, White Paper, 97
Better Services for the Mentally Ill, White Paper, 147–48
boundaries, 176

Brooklands Experiment, 97

Campaign for the Mentally Handicapped, 97
Care in the Community, consultative document, 150
Care Orders, 41–5
case conferences, and child abuse, 25; and elderly, 26
Certificate in Social Service, 101
change, 3, 19–23, 29, 86, 175
Charter of Rights for Children in Care, 27, 28
Child Care Act 1980: S1, 36; S2, 36, 37, 38, 39; S2(2), 37; S2(3), 37; S3, 36, 39, 41, 44; S3(1), 41; S3(6), 40; S4, 40; S5(2), 40; S10(1), 43; S18(1), 38; S18(3), 43; S19, 43
childhood, 66–7, 68, 86, 90
children, 5, 10, 29, 31, 59, 63–93; and handicap, 94–116; legal provisions for, 35–45; and care orders, 41–5; and reviews, 36, 43, 66, 76, 83–4
Children and Young Persons Act 1933: S44, 41, 43; Schedule I, 42
Children and Young Persons Act 1963, 97
Children and Young Persons Act 1969: S1, 43; S1(1), 41, 43; S1(2), 41; S2(4), 42; S2(12), 43; S7(7)(a), 41; S20(1), 42; S20(3), 44; S21(1), 44; S21(2), 42, 43; S22(4), 42; S23(1), 42; S27(4), 43; S70(1), 43

choice, 4, 75, 82–3, 120–26, 129, 130
Church of England Children's Society, 21
Committee on Nursing, Report, 98
communication, 4
community, 23, 88, 94, 108, 112–16
community based services, 150, 152, 163
community care, 6–9, 96–9, 103–04, 106, 115, 121–24, 147–48, 150, 151, 170
community links, 87–8
community physician, 53
compulsory powers, Chapter 2, *passim* 35–55; and elderly, 131; and mentally ill, 162
Continuing Care Project, 143–44
continuity, 19–23, 67, 77, 88, 107, 109, 111–14, 143–44
continuum of care, 23, 107, 115, 120–26
control, 63, 75, 81, 82
cost-effectiveness, 126
Court Report, 94–5, 98, 101
crisis, 29, 85
Crown Court, 44
Curtis Report, 87

death, 23, 64, 117, 145
decision making, 24–8, 30, 107, 108, 109, 110–11, 138–39, 145, 156, 158–63, 164–69
denial, 70, 72
departure, 19, 32, 75–6, 107, 111–13
dependence, 137
disability, 94–5
Disability Alliance, 122
disabled people, 5, 6
Disablement Resettlement Officer. 166

discharge, automatic, 35, 36, 47–50; by competent authority, 35, 36–45, 50–2, 53–4
District Handicap Teams, 99, 101, 108
domiciliary services, 118, 121, 127
drift, 67

Education Act 1970, 98
Education Act 1976, 101
elderly, 5, 6, 7, 8, 10, 59, 117–45; and legal provisions, 52–4
Ely Hospital, Cardiff, 97, 98
emergency, 4, 91, 133–34
empathy, 68, 70
environment, 94, 100, 102, 104, 109, 137, 140
EXODUS, 104

family, 20; and children, 71, 75, 76, 79, 85, 86–7, 88, 89; and handicapped children, 94–6, 101–03, 105, 108–09, 111, 113–16; and elderly, 127–28; case examples, 159–71
fantasy, 68, 70, 72, 80, 86
finality, 87–8
flexibility, 113, 119, 127
foster care, 8, 31, 64, 67, 72, 73, 87, 89, 106, 112, 114–15

goals, 30, 108–09, 115, 174
group living, 65, 70
groups, 80–1, 89, 90
Guardianship of Minors Act 1971, 41; S5, 40

handicapped children, 30, 59–60, 94–116
Hester Adrian Centre, 98, 103
High Court, 40, 42
holidays, 105–06, 108–09, 112–14

home help service, 119
homeless people, 21–2
hope, 63, 66, 67, 72, 90, 134
Hospital Plan, 147
hospitals, 29, 31, 32, 59, 62; and
  children, 64; and handicapped
  children, 97–101, 104, 106,
  108–10, 112, 114–15; and
  elderly, 23, 25, 30, 117; and
  mentally ill, 146–78
hostels, for children, 64, 89; for
  mentally ill, 148, 169, 171; for
  homeless, 5, 21–2

idealization, 90
identity, 73–4, 76–81, 86, 90
income, 31, 129
independence, 16, 31, 124, 129
informal care, 114, 116, 119,
  127–28
innovations, 126–27
institutionalization, 14–16, 31,
  115, 122–23, 131–32, 149,
  151–52, 169
interdependence, 71, 72
isolation, 118, 125, 133

Jay Action Group, 104
Jay Report, 101
joint funding, 150
Juvenile Court, and child's
  welfare, 40; and S3 resolution,
  40; and Care Orders, 41, 43

Kent Community Care Project,
  115, 141
key worker, 27, 60, 66, 71, 76,
  79, 80, 83, 85, 88, 90, 91, 93,
  169

legal provisions, for children,
  35–45; for mentally
  disordered, 45–52, 146; for
  elderly, 52–4
liberating education, 81, 84
local authorities, and children,

36; and discharge of Care
  Order, 43; and child's
  rehabilitation, 39, 43; and
  handicapped children, 97–8,
  104
Local Authority Social Services
  Act, 97
lodgings, 67, 69
*London Borough of Lewisham
  v. Lewisham Juvenile Court
  Justices*, 37–8
loneliness, 133
long-stay patients, 23, 108, 115,
  148, 168
loss, 9, 19–20, 85, 109, 111, 122,
  131

Magistrates' Courts Act 1980,
  40, 42
mastery, 27, 66, 67, 70, 72, 74, 90
maturity, 31
meals on wheels, 119
medical model, 154, 155
Mental Health Act 1959, 39, 45,
  47, 148; S25, 47; S26, 48, 49;
  S29, 47; S30, 46; S31(4)(5), 51;
  S41(5), 51; S43(6), 51; S47(3),
  50; S49, 50; S52(3)(d), 50; S60,
  47, 49; S63(4), 51; S65, 49;
  S123(1), 51
Mental Health (Amendment)
  Bill, 45
Mental Health Review Tribunal,
  49, 50–2
mental hospitals, 10, 11, 21, 24,
  61, 146–72
mental illness, 6, 7, 19, 146–72
mentally disordered, and
  discharge, 45–52; as voluntary
  patients, 45–7; as detailed
  patients, 47–51
milieu therapy, 154, 155
misplacement, 123–24
mobility, 129
modelling, 90
motivation, 70, 71, 72

National Assistance Act 1948,
    S47, 52–4
National Assistance
    (Amendment) Act 1951, S1(3),
    54
National Children's Bureau, 65
National Children's Homes, 65
National Development Group
    for the Mentally Handicapped,
    98
National Society for Mentally
    Handicapped Children, 97
nearest relative, 50, 51
NIMROD, 104
normalization, 103
Northgate Hospital,
    Northumberland, 103
nurse, 151, 153, 154, 155, 158,
    159, 161, 166, 167, 169

occupation, 129
outcomes, 16–18, 64, 71, 93

parents, 36–45, 64, 66, 71, 73,
    76, 77, 78, 79, 85, 87, 93, 94,
    102–03, 105–15; and
    reception into care, 37–8; and
    separation, 36; and parental
    rights resolution, 39–41
parental rights, and reception
    into care, 37–8; and S3
    resolution, 39
Parental Rights Resolution, 35,
    36–41; appeals against, 40;
    and counter-notice, 40; and
    application to juvenile court,
    40; rescission of, 40;
    termination of, 40–1
participation, 66, 74, 81–6, 129,
    158, 164, 170
planning, 14, 24–5, 26, 28–34,
    63, 66, 68, 70, 71, 73, 74–5,
    76, 82, 83, 86, 107, 108, 112,
    133–39, 144–45, 147, 150,
    156, 162, 165
Platt Report, 97

policy, 6–9, 96–9, 101, 108, 113,
    115, 147–51, 154, 176–77
Portage Project, 103
powerlessness, 66, 72, 75, 85
precipitators, 133–34
preparation, 13, 26, 31, 63, 66,
    67, 68, 70, 71, 73, 75–6,
    86–93, 107, 111–13
pressure groups, 97
priorities, 6–9
prisons, 5, 7, 12, 15, 22, 24, 31,
    32, 33
probability, 9
process of leaving, 11–34
professionals, 103, 116
psychiatrist, 151, 153, 154, 156,
    158, 159, 161, 162, 164, 165,
    166, 169
psychogeriatrics, 123
psychologist, 153, 154, 155, 158,
    159, 166
psychology, 155
punishment, 85, 86

radical residential child care,
    81–2
reality, 68, 70, 71, 72, 80,
    84
records, 79–80, 84
rehabilitation, 15, 17, 39, 43, 61,
    64, 139–43, 148, 152, 153,
    155, 167, 170
rehabilitation unit, 165
release, 16
reminiscence, 70, 72, 77, 78,
    136
resettlement, 148, 152, 170
resistance, 70, 71, 72
responsible medical officer, 49,
    50, 51
resources, 98–9, 108–09, 113
review, 30–1; and children, 36,
    43, 66, 76, 83–4; and
    handicapped children, 107,
    109–10; and elderly, 139–43,
    145

rights, of children, 67; of elderly, 119, 128–32
risk, 3, 9–10, 21, 87, 88, 89, 109, 110, 129–30, 132, 133, 137–38
role negotiation, 157, 158, 164
role play, 83, 90
runaway children, 64, 67, 84–6

sanctuary, 15
security, 18
self-care capacity, 118, 123, 135
separation, 71, 72, 76, 85
service integration, 149, 163, 170
shared living, 81
Sheldon Report, 99
sheltered housing, 124–26, 131, 141–43
short-term care, and handicapped children, 112; and elderly, 132–33
siblings, 63, 77, 89, 102, 104–06
sick role, 151, 163, 169, 170
skills, 87, 89, 90, 91–2, 111, 135–37, 140–41
South Glamorgan, 104
special schools, 95, 98–101

stress, 65–6, 68, 85
substitute family, 64, 76, 88, 106 108
survival, 66, 67, 72, 74, 90

team work, 24–5, 61, 99, 108, 139–40, 143, 155, 156–58, 159, 164–69
time, 3, 29, 67, 70, 77, 86, 173–75
token economy, 155
total institution, 122–23, 151
toy libraries, 102–03, 114
treatment, 15, 61, 153–55, 157, 166, 169

unemployment, 22, 75
unitary approach, 107, 111

voluntary child care organizations, 65, 89

Warnock Report, 100
Wessex Regional Health Authority, Care Evaluation Team, 99, 103

www.ingramcontent.com/pod-product-compliance
Ingram Content Group UK Ltd.
Pitfield, Milton Keynes, MK11 3LW, UK
UKHW020412010325
455677UK00029B/867